Overcoming Common Problems Series

Coping with Memory Problems
Dr Sallie Baxendale

Coping with Obsessive Compulsive Disorder
Professor Kevin Gournay, Rachel Piper
and Professor Paul Rogers

Coping with Phobias and Panic
Professor Kevin Gournay

Coping with Polycystic Ovary Syndrome
Christine Craggs-Hinton

Coping with the Psychological Effects of Cancer
Professor Robert Bor, Dr Carina Eriksen
and Ceilidh Stapelkamp

Coping with the Psychological Effects of Illness
Dr Fran Smith, Dr Carina Eriksen
and Professor Robert Bor

Coping with Radiotherapy
Dr Terry Priestman

Coping with Schizophrenia
Professor Kevin Gournay and Debbie Robson

Coping with Snoring and Sleep Apnoea
Jill Eckersley

Coping with Stomach Ulcers
Dr Tom Smith

Coping with Suicide
Maggie Helen

Coping with Thyroid Disease
Mark Greener

Coping with Type 2 Diabetes
Susan Elliot-Wright

Depressive Illness: The curse of the strong
Dr Tim Cantopher

The Diabetes Healing Diet
Mark Greener and Christine Craggs-Hinton

Dying for a Drink
Dr Tim Cantopher

The Empathy Trap: Understanding antisocial personalities
Dr Jane McGregor and Tim McGregor

Epilepsy: Complementary and alternative treatments
Dr Sallie Baxendale

The Fibromyalgia Healing Diet
Christine Craggs-Hinton

Fibromyalgia: Your treatment guide
Christine Craggs-Hinton

A Guide to Anger Management
Mary Hartley

Hay Fever: How to beat it
Dr Paul Carson

The Heart Attack Survival Guide
Mark Greener

Helping Children Cope with Grief
Rosemary Wells

Helping Elderly Relatives
Jill Eckersley

The Holistic Health Handbook
Mark Greener

How to Beat Worry and Stress
Dr David Delvin

How to Develop Inner Strength
Dr Windy Dryden

How to Eat Well When You Have Cancer
Jane Freeman

How to Live with a Control Freak
Barbara Baker

How to Lower Your Blood Pressure: And keep it down
Christine Craggs-Hinton

How to Manage Chronic Fatigue
Christine Craggs-Hinton

How to Stop Worrying
Dr Frank Tallis

The IBS Healing Plan
Theresa Cheung

Invisible Illness: Coping with misunderstood conditions
Dr Megan A. Arroll and Professor Christine P. Dancey

The Irritable Bowel Diet Book
Rosemary Nicol

Living with Angina
Dr Tom Smith

Living with Autism
Fiona Marshall

Living with Bipolar Disorder
Dr Neel Burton

Living with Complicated Grief
Professor Craig A. White

Living with Crohn's Disease
Dr Joan Gomez

Living with Eczema
Jill Eckersley

Living with Fibromyalgia
Christine Craggs-Hinton

Living with Gluten Intolerance
Jane Feinmann

Living with Hearing Loss
Dr Don McFerran, Lucy Handscomb
and Dr Cherilee Rutherford

Living with IBS
Nuno Ferreira and David T. Gillanders

Living with Loss and Grief
Julia Tugendhat

Livin
Dr Jo

Livin
Profe

Overcoming Common Problems Series

Living with Tinnitus and Hyperacusis
Dr Laurence McKenna, Dr David Baguley
and Dr Don McFerran

Losing a Parent
Fiona Marshall

**Making Sense of Trauma: How to tell
your story**
Dr Nigel C. Hunt and Dr Sue McHale

Menopause in Perspective
Philippa Pigache

Motor Neurone Disease: A family affair
Dr David Oliver

The Multiple Sclerosis Diet Book
Tessa Buckley

Natural Treatments for Arthritis
Christine Craggs-Hinton

Overcome Your Fear of Flying
Professor Robert Bor, Dr Carina Eriksen
and Margaret Oakes

Overcoming Anorexia
Professor J. Hubert Lacey, Christine Craggs-Hinton
and Kate Robinson

Overcoming Emotional Abuse
Susan Elliot-Wright

Overcoming Fear: With mindfulness
Deborah Ward

**Overcoming Gambling: A guide for problem
and compulsive gamblers**
Philip Mawer

Overcoming Hurt
Dr Windy Dryden

Overcoming Jealousy
Dr Windy Dryden

Overcoming Loneliness
Alice Muir

**Overcoming Panic and Related Anxiety
Disorders**
Margaret Hawkins

Overcoming Procrastination
Dr Windy Dryden

Overcoming Shyness and Social Anxiety
Dr Ruth Searle

Overcoming Stress
Professor Robert Bor, Dr Carina Eriksen
and Dr Sara Chaudry

Overcoming Worry and Anxiety
Dr Jerry Kennard

**The Pain Management Handbook:
Your personal guide**
Neville Shone

The Panic Workbook
Dr Carina Eriksen, Professor Robert Bor
and Margaret Oakes

**Physical Intelligence: How to take charge of
your weight**
Dr Tom Smith

Reducing Your Risk of Dementia
Dr Tom Smith

**Self-discipline: How to get it and how to
keep it**
Dr Windy Dryden

The Self-Esteem Journal
Alison Waines

Sinusitis: Steps to healing
Dr Paul Carson

Stammering: Advice for all ages
Renée Byrne and Louise Wright

Stress-related Illness
Dr Tim Cantopher

The Stroke Survival Guide
Mark Greener

Ten Steps to Positive Living
Dr Windy Dryden

**Therapy for Beginners: How to get the best
out of counselling**
Professor Robert Bor, Sheila Gill and Anne Stokes

Think Your Way to Happiness
Dr Windy Dryden and Jack Gordon

**Tranquillizers and Antidepressants: When to
take them, how to stop**
Professor Malcolm Lader

**Transforming Eight Deadly Emotions
into Healthy Ones**
Dr Windy Dryden

The Traveller's Good Health Guide
Dr Ted Lankester

Treating Arthritis Diet Book
Margaret Hills

Treating Arthritis: The drug-free way
Margaret Hills and Christine Horner

Treating Arthritis: More ways to a drug-free life
Margaret Hills

Treating Arthritis: The supplements guide
Julia Davies

Understanding Obsessions and Compulsions
Dr Frank Tallis

Understanding Traumatic Stress
Dr Nigel Hunt and Dr Sue McHale

**Understanding Yourself and Others:
Practical ideas from the world of coaching**
Bob Thomson

When Someone You Love Has Dementia
Susan Elliot-Wright

**When Someone You Love Has Depression:
A handbook for family and friends**
Barbara Baker

Overcoming Common Problems

Living with Fibromyalgia

Third edition

CHRISTINE CRAGGS-HINTON

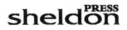

First published in Great Britain in 2000

Sheldon Press
36 Causton Street
London SW1P 4ST
www.sheldonpress.co.uk

Reprinted six times
Second edition published 2010
Reprinted four times
Third edition published 2014

British Library Cataloguing-in-Publication Data
A catalogue record for this book is available from the British Library

ISBN 978–1–84709–347–9
eBook ISBN 978–1–84709–348–6

Typeset by Fakenham Prepress Solutions, Fakenham, Norfolk NR21 8NN
First printed in Great Britain by Ashford Colour Press
Subsequently digitally reprinted in Great Britain

eBook by Fakenham Prepress Solutions, Fakenham, Norfolk NR21 8NN

Produced on paper from sustainable forests

This book is dedicated to my husband, David, and to my late father, Ernest Chamberlain.

Without the love, support and encouragement of David I would not be the 'together' person I am today, neither would I have had the confidence to research and write a book such as this.

Without my father's enduring sense of fun and determination to make the most of his lot – even in the worst days of his own illness – I would not have had the example that has helped me to cope with my fibromyalgia.

Contents

Foreword   xi

Note to the reader   xii

Introduction   xiii

1   Fibro what?   1

2   All part of the syndrome   15

3   Medication   33

4   Diet and the digestive system   42

5   Posture and exercise   58

6   Complementary therapies   88

7   Pain and stress management   110

Useful addresses   160

Further reading   164

Index   165

Foreword

Living successfully with fibromyalgia is a very difficult balancing act that requires careful management. We can now benefit from Christine's experience and knowledge, so that we do not have to spend our precious time on research.

Because medical research into fibromyalgia has made advances in the last few years, more medical professionals are now recognizing the symptoms. However, there are still many who lack the knowledge to diagnose and treat the condition effectively – and at present there are no national guidelines for treatment. That is one reason why this book is so vital to those with fibromyalgia, their families, friends and employers.

Fibromyalgia is different for each person and each person's circumstances vary, so there is no one predetermined solution. You will need to experiment with what works best for you in each area of your life.

Although self-management is crucial, it is essential that medications and supplement changes are discussed with a medical professional as combinations or sudden withdrawal can be detrimental.

There is no magic wand to make the pain disappear and restore energy levels, but there are plenty of strategies that will help. This will mean major changes in your life and could even bring about positive results that you would never have dreamed possible. The only person that can make this work is you, but *Living with Fibromyalgia* will certainly help you along the way.

Pam Stewart MBE, Chair, Fibromyalgia Association UK

Note to the reader

This is not a medical book and is not intended to replace advice from your doctor. Consult your pharmacist or doctor if you believe you have any of the symptoms described, and if you think you might need medical help.

Introduction

Fibromyalgia syndrome (FMS, for short) is a complicated condition, comprising a whole plethora of symptoms, including:

- fatigue
- insomnia
- stiffness
- anxiety
- migraines
- irritable bowel syndrome
- irritable bladder
- allergies
- depression
- cold intolerance
- dry eyes
- numbness.

The chief characteristic, however, is that of chronic, widespread soft tissue pain. In some people this pain is little more than a nagging inconvenience, but for others it is an all-consuming stabbing or burning which makes it difficult to concentrate, and that is so debilitating you can barely move without aggravating it.

Until the last decade or so, people with fibromyalgia were told they either had arthritis (despite the absence of joint inflammation) or were suffering from psychological problems. Fortunately, the medical world is now slowly acknowledging the existence of fibromyalgia, and currently more and more people are being diagnosed every day, which comes as a great relief. To be told there is a real physical reason for the persistent pain and miscellany of other symptoms is heartening. Prior to diagnosis, many people with fibromyalgia worry that their problems are of the mind rather than the body – a feeling that is compounded by negative test results. Family and friends, running short on patience and understanding, may even have begun urging, 'Try to pull yourself together!' Other people with fibromyalgia may have been convinced they were stricken with a terrible degenerative disease that, if not proving fatal, will eventually render them unable to function.

I have fibromyalgia myself and well remember the feelings of relief I experienced at my own diagnosis. It seemed as though I had finally come to the end of a long journey that had begun, eight years earlier, with a whiplash injury. I had spent all that time in constant pain, sleeping badly and feeling drained of energy. Now that, at last, my doctors knew what ailed me, I assumed they would be able to prescribe the appropriate medication. Before I knew it, I'd be back at work and getting on with my life. I couldn't have been more wrong, though. I soon learned that there are pills that lessen the symptoms, pills that make life a little more tolerable, but, sadly, no quick and simple cure-all.

As I began the task of collecting information on fibromyalgia and its related treatments, I realized I was at the start of yet another long journey. This became a journey of trial and error, of frustration and sometimes desperation. However, it has proved to be rewarding, too. Very. I am now far less debilitated than in the early days. The pain used to be so excruciating I was almost permanently bed-bound, my back and neck virtually rigid with spasm. My husband had to wash me, feed me and even brush my teeth. Now, though, because I have taken every opportunity to help myself, I am generally able to spend two hours, quite happily, at my computer; I can perform a few light tasks around the house, and I can take a short walk most days. Best of all, I can have nights out with my husband, which pleases him no end!

Admittedly, my life is still limited and I have to remember always to pace myself. I still have days when I feel like caving in under the pressure of it all, but I remind myself that I am slowly making headway – and that is a great motivator. Your health can improve, too. Indeed, if you arm yourself with knowledge – and with the impetus and encouragement that brings – your condition will, in all probability, never be as bad as it was beforehand. You should make a steady improvement and see that, once more, life can be thoroughly enjoyed.

> There is no knowledge that is not power.
> *Ralph Waldo Emerson*

1

Fibro what?

To be in constant pain; to feel too sapped to lift a limb, and to be bombarded, at the same time, by a whole host of other ailments ... that's fibromyalgia!

Although we are learning more and more about the causes of fibromyalgia, it remains a difficult condition to diagnose. No one can see the pain, and it doesn't show itself in X-rays or available blood tests and bone scans. You may have undergone a whole gamut of 'investigations', and while it is reassuring when major illnesses are ruled out, you have probably prayed, at the same time, for *something* to show up.

It may help to know that, prior to diagnosis, your doctor, likely as not, felt as mystified as you. Ironically, your doctor's inability to determine the cause of your symptoms may have been hampered by his or her medical training. Medical students learn that specific conditions produce distinctive symptoms and that elimination of the cause ensures, in most cases, full recovery. This 'classical medical model' has been used successfully for many years, leading to numerous advances in modern medicine. Unfortunately, because the difficulties presented by fibromyalgia patients do not fit this model, delayed diagnosis is common.

On a more positive note, doctors are slowly but surely familiarizing themselves with the peculiar nature of fibromyalgia and referring their patients to a rheumatologist who is familiar with the condition. A diagnosis of fibromyalgia should only be made when all other diseases are ruled out. It can therefore be said that fibromyalgia is a diagnosis of exclusion.

What is fibromyalgia?

You may wonder how the name 'fibromyalgia' came into being. The word can be split into parts that are easier to understand. 'Fibro' means fibrous connective tissue – tendons and ligaments – 'my' means muscle, and 'algia' means pain. The word 'syndrome' means a collection of symptoms that, when they occur together, identify an illness. The symptoms commonly occurring with fibromyalgia include persistent, widespread pain, fatigue, sleep disturbance, anxiety, irritable bowel problems, irritable bladder problems, reactive depression, headaches, allergies, 'foggy brain' and morning stiffness (see Chapter 2).

First the good news ... fibromyalgia is not a degenerative disease, it does not cause deformity and you are not going to die from it. Studies have shown that the majority of people with it either stay the same or improve – and, although progress is generally slow, the changes can be dramatic. However, notable advances appear only to be made in those who take steps to help themselves.

Fibromyalgia is, without doubt, a 'challenging' condition, for, as well as currently being incurable, its chief characteristic is pain. Those who have fibromyalgia often complain that they 'hurt all over', although the neck, shoulders – generally in the region between the shoulder blades – chest, lower back and buttocks seem to be the principal areas affected. The pain is mainly muscular for most people, but the tendons and ligaments are often a source of pain, too. Trapped nerves from bunched muscles can also cause pain – and this is usually a sharper, more intense pain than that coming directly from the muscles, tendons and ligaments.

Due to nearby tense and painful tissues, joint mobility is occasionally reduced in fibromyalgia – but the joints themselves don't sustain damage. There is, however, an increased risk of developing premature osteoporosis – where the bones become brittle and more prone to fractures. Post-menopausal women whose activity levels are greatly limited are at greater risk of osteoporosis than anyone else.

Widespread pain

The pain of fibromyalgia is commonly described as 'widespread', and generally arises at neuromuscular junctions – that is, the places where the muscles receive electrical input from the nerve endings. Several areas may hurt at one time, but one particular region may be the cause of most concern. Also, the pain can migrate from area to area. One day your neck may hurt so badly you can barely turn your head; the next, although your neck pain has mysteriously eased, your legs ache so much that walking is difficult.

Such bizarre comings and goings of pain are difficult to rationalize, almost impossible for onlookers to comprehend and incredibly frustrating all round. Besides often being random, the pain may fluctuate during the course of each day. Factors particular to each person can be responsible for aggravating it.

Stress is one of the greatest enemies of someone with fibromyalgia, as is the lack of restorative sleep, cold and/or humid weather conditions and too much or the wrong type of activity. Any one of these elements may provoke a flare-up of symptoms lasting for days, weeks or even months. On the other hand, symptoms can improve for no apparent reason.

Just as no two people are exactly alike, no two people with fibromyalgia experience precisely the same pain. One person may complain of searing, burning pains, another of throbbing sensations, another of tingling and numbness, and another of constant, nagging aches. Whatever the sensation felt, it is far from pleasant, and when accompanied by a multitude of other symptoms and illnesses, it is no wonder people can feel overwhelmed.

Pain origins

Pain from the following sources contributes to the overall picture.

- *Pain from muscle tension* Muscle tension creates an increased demand for blood and oxygen, yet inhibits the drainage of waste materials. This creates more pain, therefore more muscle tension (see below).
- *Pain from low muscle endurance* Sustained activity creates many difficulties in fibromyalgia. For example, you may be able to lift, in turn, three 1 kg bags of sugar without immediate pain, but shortly afterwards your muscles may begin to hurt. Lifting no more than one or two bags of sugar would, in this instance, be recommended. If you need to lift three or more bags in total, allow your muscles to rest for a few minutes between each exertion.
- *Myofascial (localized) pain* This often very acute pain is induced by 'trigger points' that are regularly 'activated' (see below).
- *Pain from microtraumas* Microtraumas are slow-healing microscopic tears in the muscle tissue. Experts believe they occur in most cases of fibromyalgia (for more details, see Chapter 2).
- *Pain from abnormal stiffness* Extreme stiffness sometimes occurs in fibromyalgia. It can arise when the individual sits or lies down for prolonged periods of time (for more details, see Chapter 2).

Pain from muscle tension

Certain muscle groups are, in all people with fibromyalgia, permanently tense and therefore painful. The tension may be due to over-activity, emotional stress or postural problems. Permanently tense muscles demand increased blood and oxygen supplies, but, at the same time, drainage of waste materials is inhibited by the tension. This leads to further tension and so further pain. The muscles eventually adapt to this cycle by becoming shorter and more fibrous, like the stringy bits in a piece of tough meat.

Gradually, these shorter, less elastic muscles begin to pull on their tendons – the structures that anchor them to the bones. The tendons then start the same process, becoming deprived of oxygen and clogged with waste materials. Like the affected muscles, they, in turn, grow fibrous and painful – and painful tissues burn energy at a terrific rate.

These tense and fibrous muscles go on to cause further problems, as, for every set of tense muscles, there is always an opposing set of weak muscles. For example, a person with weak abdominal muscles invariably has tight lower back muscles. Each set of permanently tense and fibrous muscles has an opposite set of muscles that is permanently weakened, and this eventually leads to the postural changes that typify fibromyalgia (see Figure 1).

Trigger points

Not to be confused with the 'tender points' used to diagnose fibromyalgia (see under 'Diagnosis' later in this chapter), trigger points are localized areas of pain and sensitivity occurring in permanently tense and fibrous tissues. Due to inadequate local circulation, these areas suffer from increased energy consumption and reduced oxygen supply.

When pressed, a trigger point will radiate pain and/or numbness into further areas. When 'activated' by cold, stress, over-exertion and so on, a trigger point will automatically transmit pain and numbness to further areas. If your doctor pressed a certain point on your upper back, say, and, as a result, you felt pain or numbness down one arm, the spot that was pressed would have been a trigger point.

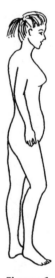

Figure 1
Postural
changes
typical of
fibromyalgia

Light-pressure, trigger-point massage generally reduces the pain and relaxes the muscle. Pain from active trigger points is a feature of almost all chronic (long-lasting) pain conditions.

Myofascial pain syndrome

You may be surprised to learn that many people with fibromyalgia also have a condition called myofascial pain syndrome (MPS for short) – I, for one, do. MPS arises from referred trigger-point pain, which occurs when one or more trigger points are regularly 'activated' (see 'Trigger points' above). It causes the localized, and often very severe, pain that is usually the worst part of our fibromyalgia. My myofascial pain is in my neck, shoulders and upper back. Other common areas are the chest, buttocks and lower back.

MPS is diagnosed in the same way as fibromyalgia (see under 'Diagnosis' later in this chapter). The following four points, taken together, can indicate the existence of MPS:

1 the presence of chronic, localized pain;
2 the fact that there is no obvious cause of the pain – that is, joint strain or arthritis;
3 the fact that the pain has responded neither to treatments prescribed for what was originally thought to be the problem, nor to further treatments, including rest;
4 the fact that the pain intensifies when you are under some kind of stress, such as after physical activity, emotional stress or exposure to cold.

There are some people, however, who have MPS and not fibromyalgia. These people experience less morning stiffness, less fatigue and less incidence of digestive disorders. The best treatment of MPS is trigger-point massage and manipulation, and fortunately more and more physiotherapists are being trained to do this. On a short-term basis, trigger points respond well to heat treatments and acupuncture.

What causes fibromyalgia?

Fibromyalgia is believed to arise from a variety of factors working together. Indeed, the following abnormalities have been found:

- *The central nervous system (the brain and spinal cord)* Advanced scanning technology has shown that people with fibromyalgia have reduced blood flow and energy production in the regions of the brain dealing with pain regulation, memory and concentration.

- *The endocrine system (the hormones)* Research into the endocrine system has shown that hormonal imbalances play a leading role in fibromyalgia. Research is now focusing on hormonal neurotransmitters.
- *The immune system (antibody protection against infection)* Immune system disturbances resulting from an overload of environmental toxins (pesticides, aerosols, car fumes and so on) and/or viral activity can arise when activated by specific triggers.

Researchers have suggested that fibromyalgia is linked to the following:

- An imbalance in the chemical serotonin, which results in lowered pain tolerance and an unrestful sleep cycle. Low serotonin levels also cause the individual to be less physically active, and the muscles and other tissues to be more sensitive, painful and easily irritated. This results in oversensitive nerve cells, often leading to widespread soft tissue pain.
- An imbalance in the chemicals cortisol and growth hormone – the release of which is controlled by the pituitary gland and hypothalamus – causing fatigue, mood changes, poor concentration and short-term memory results. An imbalance can also cause a lowered tolerance to pain and other fibromyalgia symptoms.
- Disruption of alpha-wave sleep, which results in less growth hormone being manufactured by the body (growth hormone is largely produced during this deep phase of sleep). Disturbed sleep is believed to be both a cause and an effect of fibromyalgia.
- Immune system disturbances resulting from an overload of environmental toxins – i.e. pesticides, aerosols, car fumes, food additives and preservatives, etc.

Triggers for fibromyalgia

The onset of fibromyalgia has been linked to the following triggers:

- A viral illness such as the flu or glandular fever

- A neck injury (whiplash injuries are thought to be the chief trigger of fibromyalgia)
- Surgery
- Emotional trauma and stress.

Chronic pain development

For many years, it was supposed that the same pain stimulus – such as a pinprick – produced the same degree of pain in every man, woman and child. However, we now know that if the pain stimulus is repeated many times there is an *amplification* of perceived pain, which causes the central nervous system (CNS, for short) to become sensitized. (The primary function of the CNS, located in the brain and spinal cord, is to analyse input from nerve cells.)

In 1992, researchers found that persistent severe pain will only arise in an individual who has suffered severe pain in the past (the CNS 'remembers' past pain intensity) and only after physical trauma, such as an injury or surgery, when the person concerned limits movement of the affected area. The individual expects to feel better after limiting movement, but many find that their pain levels have actually increased. We see, therefore, how persistent pain can arise.

Persistent pain can quite easily advance into a chronic pain situation – the second step towards central sensitization. In fact, modern scanning technology has demonstrated that pro-longed pain can create a gradual build-up of electrical response throughout the CNS. The currents can build to such intensity that a state of chronic pain results – where the CNS is sensitized to pain. All chronic pain conditions involve a degree of central sensitization. Indeed, the central nervous systems of some people are so sensitive that they experience excruciating pain when per-forming the simplest of activities.

My own pain levels invariably increase after I have inflicted a series of physical traumas on my body – such as spending too long on the computer for a few days in succession. Subsequent to an initial pain flare-up, I find that if I try to carry out the same level of activity as beforehand, the pain comes on far more easily because my pain threshold has temporarily lowered. I need to reduce my activity levels (and at the same time maintain my mobility by carrying out an exercise regime, as discussed in

Chapter 5) in order to slowly reduce the degree of central sensitization and so help myself back to my earlier state.

Medical professionals have long been bewildered by the severity of pain in fibromyalgia. Studies have shown, however, that we have very low pain thresholds – due, in part, to the effects of central sensitization. This means that we are likely to experience distinct and troublesome pain where a healthy person may only feel discomfort. Of course, this in no way signifies that people with fibromyalgia are 'soft' or 'weak', for evidence suggests that we complain far less than the average person.

Neck trauma

Research conducted in 1997 suggests that physical trauma to the neck area is associated with a high risk of developing fibromyalgia. Dan Buskila, an Israeli doctor, compared the progress of patients with soft tissue neck injuries (usually occurring after whiplash) with patients who had leg fractures. He found that, after approximately three months, fibromyalgia is 13 times more likely to develop following a neck injury than a lower extremity injury.

The difference may be due to the fact that the area injured in whiplash (the dorsal horn) plays an important role in filtering pain signals to the brain. Some experts believe that trauma to this area can severely impair the filtering mechanisms, allowing the pain-processing centre in the CNS to be bombarded with pain messages. They are of the opinion that such localized post-traumatic malfunction can gradually evolve into the widespread pain disorder that is fibromyalgia (see 'Chronic pain development' above). Many researchers are, as a result, focusing on the pain-filtering mechanisms within the dorsal horn.

Spinal abnormalities

At the 1997 FMS International Conference, Professor W. Muller presented a study suggesting that some people with fibromyalgia have structural abnormalities, occurring mostly in the cervical (neck) and lumbar (lower back) regions of the spine. Indeed, later studies using MRI (Magnetic Resonance Imaging) scans have shown that there is a higher than normal incidence of narrowing of the cervical spine canal in fibromyalgia. The malformation is known as cervical stenosis and is usually genetic in origin, i.e. the tendency to have it runs in families. Experts are theorizing that mechanical irrita-tions caused by such an abnormality can cause constant 'injury' input to the CNS, effectively leading to persistent pain and central sensitization.

When the cervical spine is narrower than normal, tilting the neck backwards can lead to spinal cord compression, which, in turn, restricts the flow of blood and spinal fluid to the CNS. Tilting the head forwards, so your chin is close to your chest, can stretch the spinal cord, causing mechanical irritation of the nerves running along it. This irritation is ultimately perceived as pain.

As most people with fibromyalgia have neck pain, activities that repeatedly flex the neck should be avoided. Instead of straining your neck, use your eyes as much as possible. Wearing a surgical collar is not recommended as it will only weaken your muscles. There is also an increased likelihood of strain once the collar is removed. Strengthening your neck muscles with exercise is, ulti-mately, the most useful advice I can offer (see Chapter 5 for neck exercises).

Abnormal hormone levels

The pain of fibromyalgia can also be provoked and amplified by abnormalities in certain body chemicals. We now know that elev-ated levels of the pain-transmitting chemical called *substance P* is one of the principal causes of severe pain in fibromyalgia, whereas low levels of the chemical *serotonin* is primarily responsible for the lack of pain control.

Substance P plays an important role in the biochemical pain sequence, for when a person experiences a painful trauma, such as a trapped finger, there is an immediate release of substance P into the spinal cord. A series of messages are then transmitted, one of which tells the brain that the finger is injured. Several studies have shown that, regardless of the triggering factor in fibromyalgia, there are abnormally high levels of substance P present in the individual's spinal fluid. This means that people with the condition experience a greater level of perceived pain than normal. Other chronic pain disorders display slight elevations of substance P, but the levels are not nearly so high as in fibromyalgia.

As mentioned on page 7, chronic pain can give rise to central sen-sitization. Fibromyalgia apparently arises when pain-transmitting chemicals – the primary one being substance P – accumulate to such an extent that they overflow from injured tissues into neighbouring healthy tissues, increasing, in turn, their sensitivity to pain. In some instances, this hormone can pervade the entire spinal cord. As a consequence, everyday activity can result in pain that, in turn, can lead to impaired function. Indeed, sensitization of erstwhile healthy tissues may even cause light touch to be experienced as pain. After doing something so seemingly insignificant as scratching a tiny itch, many people with fibromyalgia – myself included – experience acute pain in that area which lasts for several minutes.

Pain circuitry

Research conducted in 1991 by Dr Clifford Woolf suggests that altered neuron programming can add to the pain problem in fibromyalgia. There are two types of nerve fibres – nociceptive neurons and non-nociceptive neurons – multitudes of which exist alongside each other throughout the body. Normally, an injury such as a trapped finger produces distinct physical and chemical changes that are picked up by nociceptive neurons. Messages are rapidly relayed between the finger and the CNS, one of which creates the consciousness of localized pain. (The same series of events takes place with all peripheral injuries – a broken arm, cut knee, stubbed toe or whatever.) The non-nociceptive nerve fibres in the injured area are not normally involved in the pain process. These fibres relay only tactile-type messages to the CNS such as a kiss, stroke, light massage or pat on the back. They also transmit sensations of muscle movement such as walking, raising your arms or turning your head.

When the CNS is hypersensitized (see 'Chronic pain development' above), previously innocuous non-nociceptive neurons can unfortunately be hijacked into becoming pain transmitters. Dr Woolf has, in fact, been able to show that, in chronic pain conditions, non-nociceptive neurons often alter their programming to mimic nociceptive neurons. Some are such mimics they even start releasing substance P! This is a further reason that people with fibromyalgia feel pain during or after experiences that are not 'ordinarily' painful.

It must be stated that not all chronic pain conditions hijack non-nociceptive neurons into acting as pain messengers. We can only assume that people's genetic make-up determines whether or not they will be affected.

Fine nerve abnormalities

In line with recent thinking about fibromyalgia as a disorder of the CNS involving changes in pain processing, whereby an oversensitive CNS amplifies pain messages, research is increasingly showing evidence for fine nerve damage in fibromyalgia. These peripheral nerve abnormalities could be the real reason why we are so much more sensitive to pain, and feel it more acutely.

Some research has suggested that more than half of fibromyalgia cases have evidence of actual nerve damage – evidence at last that it's not all in our minds. In 2013, neurologist Dr Anne Louise Oaklander at Massachusetts General Hospital in Boston led two studies that showed that the damage affects the fine nerves of the body. As a result, these small nerves give off faulty signals, causing many of the symptoms with which we are only too familiar in fibromyalgia – pain, sleep disturbance, digestive problems and so on.

More evidence that fibromyalgia may be a fine nerve condition comes from neuroscientist Dr Frank Rice and colleagues at Albany Medical College, who in 2013 found that people with fibromyalgia have excessive nerve fibres lining blood vessels in the skin. Women have more of these fibres than men – one reason perhaps why there are more women than men with fibromyalgia.

Work in 2012 by neuroscientist Dr Jordi Serra of the University of Barcelona and University College London also supports the idea that some people with fibromyalgia have peripheral neuropathy (damage or disease to the nerves) and that FMS is a neuropathic pain condition (pain that results from problems with nerve signals).

It's been suggested that such cases of fine nerve damage fall into another condition called small fibre peripheral neuropathy (SFPN), which can cause widespread pain.

Not all doctors agree with this – some say that fibromyalgia includes symptoms that aren't typical of SFPN, such as widespread muscle and soft tissue pain, though this doesn't rule out the possibility that similar minute nerve damage in muscles and tendons could still be to blame. Many researchers, however, such as Dr Oaklander and colleagues, feel that a correct diagnosis is important because, unlike fibromyalgia, some cases of SFPN have known causes which may be treatable. They argue that a diagnosis of SFPN could make doctors look harder for an underlying cause which is treatable, such as hepatitis or diabetes. Hopefully, a thorough physical examination from your doctor has ruled out other co-existing conditions, but if in doubt, it may be worth going back for a reappraisal.

Familial links

Research indicates that fibromyalgia can run in families. This may be due to either the family environment (familial exposure to the same oil/gas fumes, aerosol sprays, glue, varnish and so on) or it may be genetic in nature. In some cases, it may even be both. Preliminary evidence suggesting that the condition can indeed be inherited, particularly by the women in a family, has been found. Men have the same family genes, but their hormonal milieu appears to offer a measure of protection.

A possible rogue gene

Scientists are now speculating that the processing of painful stimuli may be regulated by a person's genetic make-up. In other words, they suspect that people with fibromyalgia may have a rogue gene, which makes their bodies react strongly to stimuli that would merely cause discomfort in an individual without the gene. Research is underway to identify such a gene, if it exists.

Who gets fibromyalgia?

Anyone can develop fibromyalgia, but, probably owing to hormonal differences, it is present in seven to ten times more women than men. The onset of the condition is usually between the ages of 30 and 50, although many children are affected, and it can arise in people aged 75 and over. Surveys in various countries point to fibromyalgia affecting between 2 and 3.2 per cent of the population, and it's believed that numerous cases have not yet been diagnosed. As the symptoms of fibromyalgia vary so much in severity, some experts believe many people have either not yet consulted a doctor or have had their health problems dismissed as anxiety, depression, neurosis and such other problems, or as symptoms of a disorder from which they are known to be suffering.

Although fibromyalgia can arise in isolation, it often develops in people who already have a pain condition such as rheumatoid arthritis, lupus or osteoarthritis.

Diagnosis

People with fibromyalgia have areas of extreme tenderness in specific locations – usually at junctions of muscle and bone. These areas are known as tender points. They may be exquisitely painful when palpated (pressed), but otherwise they may or may not cause pain.

In 1990, the American College of Rheumatology defined the official criteria for the diagnosis of fibromyalgia:

- a history of pain in both sides of the body, pain above and below the waist, pain along the spine; and
- pain or tenderness in 11 out of 18 tender points, sited at specific locations in the body (see Figure 2).

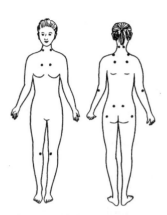

Figure 2 The 18 tender points used to establish a diagnosis of fibromyalgia

Treatment

Doctors are trained to strive to cure illness. Indeed, the gratification they experience on restoring patients to full health makes a demanding job feel worthwhile. Being able to help people is usually the reason they entered the medical profession in the first place. So what happens when patients are diagnosed with fibromyalgia, for which, currently, there is no cure?

At present, there is little doctors can do to correct the disorders that underlie fibromyalgia. Painkillers can reduce pain for a time – they usually prove invaluable in a pain flare-up – but they have no positive long-term effects. Certain antidepressants are known to go some way towards redressing the chemical imbalance of fibromyalgia, but they are unable to permanently correct it. People may even suffer adverse side effects after taking such medications for a long period. Referrals to physiotherapy are also commonplace in fibromyalgia. However, as some physiotherapists still know little or nothing of the condition, manipulation and prescribed exercise can aggravate the pain. The doctor may later refer the individual to relevant specialists dealing with the disorders connected with fibromyalgia; for example, a gastroenterologist if irritable bowel syndrome is diagnosed or an allergy clinic if allergies are an issue. Treatments for these conditions may prove beneficial, but such people can do little to minimize the main symptom – pain.

Some doctors choose to make referrals to pain or rheumatology clinics, but, again, people are invariably disappointed. Assessments are all too brief and although some may be offered painkilling injections, they are not suitable for everyone. The majority of people with fibromyalgia are dismissed feeling they haven't been taken seriously. It may help to know that what appears to be lack of interest is, in many cases, sheer frustration at being unable to do or say anything useful.

Chronic, intractable pain presented a stumbling block for the medical profession for many years. Fortunately, health authorities have now recognized the need to adopt a different approach, as a result of which pain rehabilitation programmes are already up and running at hospitals and health centres all over the UK. The programmes offer cognitive behavioural therapy – a psychotherapeutic approach that teaches a variety of pain management techniques.

At each two-hour session, the patient joins a group of people with similar problems. Working together they learn goal setting, problem solving and other cognitive behavioural skills aimed at managing the psychological difficulties that arise with chronic pain, such as stress, anxiety and mood swings. They also learn a stretching and strengthening regime tailored to their particular limitations. The programmes are normally run by senior physiotherapists, a GP and a cognitive therapist, who are joined on certain days by a pain specialist and a psychologist.

Pain rehabilitation programmes do not offer a cure, but they can mean that the individual understands more about the nature of chronic pain, is more physically active, less emotionally distressed, is able to use a range of relaxation skills and, ultimately, becomes less reliant on medication. Someone who attended the first programme at Bradford Royal Infirmary was noted as saying, 'From the beginning I realized the other patients were just like me, frustrated and in pain – and from all walks of life. We were not promised a cure, but we were going to learn how to manage our pain.'

2

All part of the syndrome

> I thought I was going out of my mind! Sleep problems, stomach problems, fatigue, a sensitivity to many of the everyday things in life – on top of the constant pain ... It was such a relief to find they were all part of the same illness!

Fibromyalgia, as we have seen, is a syndrome, which means that other conditions are associated with the disorder. These conditions may be present without fibromyalgia, but are so often seen with fibromyalgia that they are now considered a part of the syndrome. This chapter deals with the most common of these conditions, excluding soft tissue pain, which is discussed in other chapters.

Conditions typically occurring with fibromyalgia include:

- muscular pain
- fatigue
- disturbed sleep
- depression
- anxiety
- irritable bowel syndrome
- headaches
- allergies
- muscle spasms
- cognitive dysfunction ('foggy brain')

- morning stiffness
- irritable bladder
- dry eyes and mouth
- restless arms and legs
- numbness and tingling
- skin problems
- temperomandibular joint dysfunction (jaw pain).

Other possible symptoms are:

- bloated feeling (particularly in hands and feet)
  - photophobia (extreme sensitivity to light)
  - poor tolerance to extreme temperatures and humidity
- chronic rhinitis (a persistently runny nose)
- bruxism (teeth grinding during sleep)
- mouth ulcers
- bruising easily.

Fatigue

Although chronic fatigue is almost universal in fibromyalgia, in some it is barely discernible, but in others it is extreme, like the exhaustion that comes with a bad dose of flu. At times, your muscles may feel worn to their limit, even though you have just woken up. People less severely affected can find that relaxing in a chair for half an hour is enough to restore their flagging energy levels.

The best way to manage all but extreme weariness is to alternate activity with periods of rest. The key is to listen to your body. Don't try to push yourself when you feel exhausted already. It is tempting to, I know, but finishing off that pile of ironing before you flop onto the sofa will only make you feel worse.

Serotonin

Most people with fibromyalgia are known to have an abnormally low supply of serotonin – a chemical neurotransmitter that sends messages to the vital organs and interacts with substance P to determine pain levels. Medication that helps to slow down the removal of serotonin from the body – called selective serotonin re-uptake inhibitors, or SSRIs – can help to combat fatigue, depression, sleep problems and so on. Such drugs include paroxetine (Seroxat), sertraline (Lustral), fluoxetine (Prozac) and duloxetine (Cymbalta, Xeristar). Although this type of medication is classed as 'antidepressant', it is for its serotonin raising qualities that it is used in fibromyalgia. If your doctor prescribes an SSRI, carefully follow his or her directions.

Seasonal affective disorder (SAD)

During winter, the decline in daylight hours can cause a marked decrease in the amount of serotonin produced by the body, triggering an increase in fatigue, depression, anxiety and so on in individuals with fibromyalgia and other susceptible people. This phenomenon gives rise to what is now known as seasonal affective disorder (SAD), which affects an estimated half a million people in the UK each winter.

People with fibromyalgia have serotonin in low supply anyway, which goes some way towards explaining why their symptoms generally worsen in winter. Treatment to replace the availability of serotonin can take the form of light therapy – that is, exposure for up to four hours a day to very bright light, at least ten times the intensity of ordinary domestic lighting. The individual should sit 0.6–0.9 metres (2–3 feet) from a specially designed lightbox, placed perhaps on a table, where it is then possible to carry out normal activities – reading, writing, eating, knitting and so on. Provided the lightbox is used daily, benefits should be felt within three or four days, and will continue throughout the winter months. (See the Useful addresses section at the back of the book for details of lightbox sale and hire and for the address of the UK SAD Association.)

When a person with fibromyalgia uses light therapy in conjunction with medication that moderates the removal of serotonin (SSRIs), the difficulties encountered during winter months can be greatly reduced.

Hypoglycaemia

A word or two of warning: fatigue should never be presumed to be an element of fibromyalgia. Indeed, as your particular symptoms may relate to any one of numerous disorders, they should always be discussed with your doctor. For example, headaches, confusion, visual disturbance, muscle weakness, impaired muscle co-ordination and extreme mood swings should be taken very seriously as they indicate a type of hypoglycaemia. Another type of hypoglycaemia is characterized by faintness, weakness, jitteriness, nerviness and excessive hunger.

Early diagnosis of hypoglycaemia is crucial. (If left untreated, the first set of symptoms can lead to loss of consciousness, convulsions and, eventually, coma.)

Chronic fatigue syndrome (CFS)

In discussing fatigue, chronic fatigue syndrome (also called myalgic encephalomyelitis (ME)) should be mentioned, as it has many symptoms in common with fibromyalgia. However, in fibromyalgia the pain is the chief symptom whereas in CFS it is fatigue. Like fibromyalgia, CFS is a condition of exclusion – in other words, doctors need first to rule out other causes before a diagnosis can be made. A small number of fibromyalgia patients suffer from such extreme fatigue that they are also diagnosed with CFS. The treatments for CFS are very similar to fibromyalgia, and there are now several good books on the subject (see the Further reading section at the back of this book).

Sleep problems

As with muscle pain and fatigue, sleep problems appear to be present in all cases of fibromyalgia. In fact, poor sleep quality is seen as being a cause of the condition as well as a result. Due to the abnormal brain wave patterns found in fibromyalgia, most are simply unable to achieve deep, restorative sleep.

Poor sleep has long been recognized as one of the hallmarks of fibromyalgia, and in particular, brainwave studies show that loss of deep sleep is common and frequent. Research has found that in adults over 50, non-restorative sleep – the kind when you wake up feeling tired and jaded – has a strong link with widespread pain, another key symptom of fibromyalgia. Dr John McBeth and colleagues, of Keele University, Staffordshire, also found that anxiety, memory problems and poor physical health are linked to a higher risk of developing widespread pain.

In a large ten-year study published in the journal *Arthritis and Rheumatism*, researchers from Norway found a link between sleep problems and an increased risk of fibromyalgia, particularly in middle-aged and older women. Dr Tom Nilsen and Dr Paul Mork from the Norwegian University of Science and Technology studied 12,350 women and found that women from 45 years upwards who often or always had sleep problems had almost twice the risk of developing fibromyalgia as those aged between 20 and 44 years old.

It's thought that sleep disturbance may contribute to the increased sensitivity to pain and physical stimulus felt by people with fibromyalgia. Studies have repeatedly shown that healthy volunteers repeatedly woken from deep sleep developed symptoms of fibromyalgia, thus demonstrating how easily disturbed sleep may lead to a vicious cycle of severe tiredness, depression and sensitivity to pain.

Throughout sleep, the brain continues to rule the body functions by controlling the release of various hormones. The levels of prolactin and testosterone – the growth hormones – rise significantly during deep, delta-phase sleep, facilitating tissue repair and regeneration. Good health depends on an individual being able to achieve this type of restorative sleep each and every night. Wouldn't you just know it, though – the majority of people with fibromyalgia have difficulty attaining delta-phase sleep. Light, alpha-phase sleep constantly interrupts this important level, causing the individual to wake feeling almost as tired as when he or she retired the previous night.

Because delta-phase sleep is rarely achieved in fibromyalgia, most people with the condition have growth hormones in low supply. These essential hormones can, to some extent, be induced by changing to a high-protein diet, taking mineral supplements – preferably before bedtime – and using relaxation techniques (all discussed in later chapters). However, if no action is taken to replace at least some of the lost growth hormones, the lack of delta-phase sleep can cause the muscles to continue to be painful.

In 1993, a researcher was able to demonstrate how easily disturbed sleep can affect the muscles. Six volunteers (people without fibromyalgia) were, for three consecutive nights, repeatedly woken during delta-phase sleep; they all began to display the diffuse pain, fatigue and tender sites present in fibromyalgia. On the other hand, fully fit long-distance runners were unaffected after being disturbed in the same way. It can be seen, therefore, that carefully controlled lifestyle changes, involving dietary improvements, better relaxation and the careful introduction of exercise, can be very helpful in fibromyalgia.

Depression

Depression, as you can imagine, is commonly found in people with chronic pain. Wouldn't anyone become depressed if they had pain every day? Until the 1990s, depression was believed to be one of the factors leading to the development of fibromyalgia. Nowadays, it is recognized as being a reaction to the condition.

One of the most unfortunate features of fibromyalgia is its invisibility. No one can see the pain, and people tend to look blank, maybe even suspicious, when you explain that you suffer from fibromyalgia. 'Fibro what?' They have never heard of it! 'Does it mean you ache a bit from time to time? We all ache a bit! Surely you're just being soft!' This type of reaction really can trigger mild depression or emphasize that which is already present. (I will explain one or two strategies for dealing with such comments in Chapter 7.) It is advisable to concentrate on the people in your life who at least try to understand how you feel. Doing so can eliminate many negative feelings. (See Chapter 3 for details of antidepressant medication.)

Anxiety

Anxiety is widespread in fibromyalgia. As with depression, anxiety often arises as a result of being in pain, feeling constantly tired and experiencing an endless barrage of other unpleasant symptoms. People with fibromyalgia who have no choice but to limit certain activities often grow anxious before attempting something unfamiliar. The more insular the individual has become, the more difficult out-of-the-ordinary situations are for him or her to handle.

To determine anxiety, ask yourself these questions.

- Am I more easily upset than usual?
- Do I feel I am overreacting to certain situations?
- Am I unusually edgy?
- Do I find it difficult to relax?
- Am I having more trouble than usual in sleeping?
- Am I breathing more shallowly than usual?

If you can answer 'yes' to any one of these questions, you are probably suffering from anxiety. Anxiety has the effect of stimulating the sympathetic nervous system – the mechanisms in the brain that respond automatically to certain occurrences – making you more tense, more tired and, ultimately, more anxious. Learning to relax effectively is easier said than done, but as anxiety is such a distressing condition, it is worth trying to follow a regular deep breathing and relaxation routine (see Chapter 7 for details).

Relaxed muscles use far less energy than tense ones and improved breathing leads to better circulation and oxygenation, which in turn helps the muscles and connective tissues. Also, a calm, relaxed mind can greatly aid concentration and short-term memory. It can clear brain fog, too.

In order to cope with anxiety more effectively, it is advisable to either limit or cut out certain stimulants, particularly caffeine, alcohol and nicotine. Stimulants are known to exacerbate anxiety, and the aforementioned products are the chief culprits. In fact, most of the symptoms of chronic anxiety may be due to the effects of high caffeine intake alone (see Chapter 4 for further information regarding caffeine).

Panic attacks

More commonly known as the panic attack, acute hyperventilation, or overbreathing, is a common affliction in fibromyalgia. A panic attack is an emotional response to anticipated stress. Often the perceived threat is obvious, but sometimes there are no apparent reasons for the onset of panicky feelings. In the latter instance, the reason may be buried in earlier life events. Talking to a counsellor may unlock buried fears and help the individual to see them in a new, more manageable light.

As a rule, panic attacks are preceded by intensifying anxiety. The individual will start breathing faster in troubled apprehension. Light-headedness, palpitations and the sensation that the chest is tightening will then be accompanied by feelings of inadequacy, fear and maybe of impending doom.

Daily deep breathing exercises – where breathing is slowed down and, on inhalation, the abdomen (not the ribcage) is allowed to rise – are very useful training. An immediate remedy is the good old paper bag. Place the bag over your nose and mouth and try to breathe more slowly. Breathing into the bag will ensure that most of the exhaled carbon dioxide is returned to your lungs. (Correct breathing is discussed in great detail in Chapter 7.)

Irritable bowel syndrome (IBS)

Fibromyalgia is, to a large extent, a problem of muscle irritability. This fact is more obvious in the muscles under voluntary control – those of the back, shoulders, stomach, buttocks and so on – but the so-called 'smooth' muscles under involuntary control can be equally affected, giving rise to bowel and bladder problems, as well as to headaches (the latter two of which are discussed later in this chapter).

Many experts believe that irritable bowel syndrome (IBS for short) arises largely as a result of muscle irritability. Fibromyalgia and IBS do appear to be closely linked. Indeed, it appears that more than half of the people diagnosed with IBS display many of the symptoms of fibromyalgia. Further apparent links will be explained in Chapter 4, when the digestive system is discussed in greater detail.

IBS is characterized by recurrent cramping pains, together with alternating bouts of diarrhoea and constipation, but some people have just diarrhoea or just constipation. Abdominal wind, bloating, heartburn, backache, nausea and lethargy are all elements of the syndrome, too. The majority of people experience just a few of the above symptoms, but an unlucky minority have them all.

A survey conducted in 1997 by the Fibromyalgia Network, Arizona, revealed that 64 per cent of people with fibromyalgia also have IBS.

Chronic yeast infections and IBS

IBS has no single, distinct cause, but research has shown that it can develop after a severe bout of 'Spanish tummy' or gastroenteritis or after taking a course of antibiotics – prescribed, maybe, to treat the infection. Antibiotics effectively kill the micro-organisms that cause disease, but they kill friendly bacteria at the same time, causing an imbalance of gut microflora.

Friendly bacteria are essential to the well-being of the digestive system, for they not only aid digestion, they also protect against parasitic yeast infections, commonly known as thrush or candida (*candida albicans*). Indeed, candida infections were relatively unknown until the advent of antibiotics in the 1940s!

Although some practitioners remain sceptical about the role of candida in IBS, many others have found that when the infection is eliminated, the symptoms of IBS decrease. Candida growth can be encouraged by oral contraceptives (commonly known as the Pill), steroids, immuno-suppressive anti-inflammatory drugs, nutritional deficiencies, high-sugar diets and any condition that weakens the immune system (cancer and AIDS are obvious examples). (See Chapter 4 for information on candida control.)

Mercury fillings and IBS

There is a growing tide of feeling that the mercury used in dental fillings is at the root of many of today's illnesses. Some researchers are convinced that mercury leaking from amalgam fillings interferes with the immune system. They believe that instead of killing bad bacteria, the immune system, confused, begins to attack the body's own cells – the muscles and ligaments. In this situation, the immune system would then begin to set up antibodies to certain foods, thus developing food intolerance. Again we see a possible link between fibromyalgia and IBS.

Food intolerance and IBS

Whether or not there is a link between food intolerance and IBS has engendered much debate in the medical world, for whereas many natural practitioners believe food intolerance to be the underlying cause of IBS, many conventional doctors reject the theory outright.

Such diverse opinion may, in part, have arisen due to confusion between the words 'allergy' and 'intolerance'. When we discover that a certain food disagrees with us, we say we are 'allergic' to it. However, as there is generally no immunological reaction to that food – that is, if our body fails to act as if it is being invaded by a foreign body, thereby setting up 'antibody' chemicals – we are using the wrong term.

A true allergy produces anything from a streaming nose, hives or a migraine attack to an extreme, life-threatening immune response such as anaphylactic shock. Intolerance, on the other hand, is caused by a slow build-up of 'problem' foods and, unlike an allergic reaction where the backlash is immediate, the response is delayed. The body eventually becomes 'sensitized' to foods that, ironically, are often the ones we eat most, inducing anything from stomach irritation (abdominal cramps, perhaps accompanied by diarrhoea), to cravings, to indigestion, all of which are unpleasant.

An increasing body of evidence is prompting experts to believe that IBS develops as a result of food intolerance. Sadly, it would appear that, because many researchers fail to allow for the delayed response, the vital connection is missed.

The foods most likely to cause problems are wheat, corn, food colourings, coffee, yeasts, citrus fruits and dairy products, as well as foods containing chemical additives and preservatives (all processed foods, in effect). Food intolerance will always be a threat to people who fail to eat a varied diet.

A safe and mild cleansing regime – where problem foods are

excluded, then slowly reintroduced – can help to reduce food intolerance (details are given in Chapter 4).

Stress and IBS

Stress and anxiety are believed to contribute to the development
of IBS and are known to play a major role in intensifying the
symptoms. As stress can have the effect of suppressing the immune
system, the employment of stress-relieving techniques is generally
helpful in treating IBS (see Chapter 7 for more details).

Any out of the ordinary bowel activity must be reported to your
doctor. Depending on your particular symptoms, the doctor may
decide to refer you to a specialist for tests. A diagnosis of IBS is
normally made when symptoms persist and yet no specific bowel
disorder is evident. This makes it yet another disease of 'exclusion'.

Headaches

As headaches are a common symptom of many of the conditions
occurring with fibromyalgia, it is hardly surprising that, according
to one survey, 59 per cent of people with the syndrome endure
headaches regularly. Tension headaches and migraines are most
prevalent. Sometimes, however, headaches can be provoked by
a sinus infection. Your doctor should be informed of your exact
symptoms.

Tension headaches

Less intense than a migraine, tension headaches are miserable
nevertheless. Tension in the neck – from where the pain usually
originates – causes muscles to contract, giving rise to the feeling of
a tight elastic band across the affected area. Pain is often first felt at
the base of the neck, spreading upwards to the temples.

Painkillers are invaluable for all types of headaches, but they
are most effective in the early stages of pain. However, as stress no
doubt aggravates and may even be the cause of most headaches,
it is useful to learn stress-management techniques. A simple tip –
lavender essential oil, mixed as directed on the bottle with a carrier
oil, massaged into the forehead and temples can help reduce the
pain. The herb wild lettuce, when made into a tea, is also a great
curative.

Migraine

This type of acutely painful headache is characterized by one-sided intense throbbing, sensitivity to light and sound, nausea and sometimes vomiting. Attacks are caused by the constriction and dilation of the tiny capillaries that take blood to the brain and can be triggered by stress (as already indicated), anxiety, fatigue, watching TV, loud noises, flickering light and a sensitivity to such things as red wine, aged and strong cheeses, chocolate, coffee, tea, alcohol and cured meats such as hot dog sausages, salami, bacon and ham.

If you suffer from migraines, it is recommended that you keep a record of all the foods and drinks consumed in the hours preceding an attack. The triggering factors should soon become apparent.

Smokers who have regular migraine attacks would be wise to try to quit. As the nicotine in tobacco causes the blood vessels to narrow, migraine attacks are always a possibility. Regular exercise is important, too (see Chapter 5), as is eating healthily (see Chapter 4). Also, it is advisable to eat three or more small meals a day, and a meal should never be skipped. Helpful complementary therapies include homeopathy, herbal medicine, acupuncture, cranial osteopathy and reflexology (see Chapter 6).

Allergies

It is estimated that half the people with fibromyalgia also have a history of allergy (toxicity) problems. The allergenic substances may be environmental (dust or pollen) or a specific medication may be responsible. However, it is likely that some so-called 'allergic' reactions (see Chapter 4) are simply a part of the enhanced sensitivity that goes with fibromyalgia.

Chemical sensitivity

Some researchers are now of the opinion that exposure to certain chemicals (pesticides, artificial fertilizers, petro-chemical fumes, glue, varnish, aerosol sprays, some household cleaners, some paints, some perfumes ... the list is endless) in our environment, as well as exposure to certain medications, may be responsible for many of the symptoms found in both fibromyalgia and chronic fatigue syndrome. Interestingly, apart from a few exceptions, it is no coincidence that in countries with little industrial power and where fresh food is grown without chemicals and eaten straight from the land, there is generally a marked absence or low incidence of allergies.

Chemical sensitivity can give rise to profound effects, including fatigue, headaches, nausea, short-term memory loss, mood changes, and numbness and tingling in the fingers and toes. A sensitivity to certain chemicals, on the other hand, is thought to restrict blood flow to and through the parts of the brain dealing with pain regulation, memory and concentration. Furthermore, a chemically overloaded immune system may, in its growing confusion, begin to react to all manner of environmental substances – and chemically sensitive individuals are more likely than others to develop true allergies.

Dr Joe Fitzgibbon, in his book *Feeling Tired All the Time* (Gill and Macmillan, 2001), illustrates how grim chemical sensitivity can be. His wife, after chronic exposure to oil and later gas fumes, developed intense migraine attacks, nausea, vomiting, extreme exhaustion and, eventually, partial paralysis. She was ill for four years, then, after staying with friends in an all-electric house for a while, the symptoms miraculously receded. Needless to say, the couple moved into an all-electric house of their own!

Sensitization to chronic chemical exposure is now well documented. Mechanics have been known to become sensitized to petrol fumes, painters to paint, printers to ink and so on. Maybe we should all take a closer look at our immediate environments. Eliminating – or at least reducing – our particular trigger factors could greatly lessen some of the symptoms tied in with our fibromyalgia. Trigger factors are not always easy to spot, however. Many medical professionals maintain that a healthy diet, rest, relaxation and plenty of exercise can help increase the body's tolerance of chemicals.

Gulf War syndrome

Chemical sensitivity is being vigorously researched – particularly after the problems experienced by veterans of the first Gulf War as a result of the exposure to cocktails of chemicals during their tours of duty. It is interesting to note that Gulf War veterans affected with what is now called Gulf War syndrome report precisely the same symptoms as do people with fibromyalgia.

Muscle spasms

Muscle spasms are common in fibromyalgia, occurring most frequently in the back, buttocks and legs. They can be defined as involuntary muscular contractions and feel rather as if the affected area is in cramp. The muscles contract due to reduced blood flow and a resulting shortage of oxygen to the muscle tissues.

Microtrauma

Muscle microtrauma (microscopic tears in the muscle fibres) may be an additional cause of spasms. For a few days after overexertion, these small tears can leak substances that cause muscle stiffness and pain. In addition, microtrauma is believed to reduce the production of energy in the muscle, thereby causing muscle fatigue.

Experts believe there can be a great deal of muscle microtrauma in fibromyalgia, and that it occurs because of a genetic predisposition. The microtrauma can be limited by pacing yourself, increasing exercise levels at a very slow rate and stopping an activity as soon as your muscles begin to protest.

The use of cold rather than heat in treatment

Spasms can be prevented by regularly changing position and keeping as mobile as possible. The pain of a spasm can be relieved by the use of heat, massage or gentle trigger-point pressure.

Cold is an effective painkiller, too. The mere mention of the word 'cold' may cause a person with fibromyalgia to wince. Cold weather can induce a severe flare-up, so how can it relax a muscle spasm? There is a great difference between walking to the shop on a bitterly cold day, however, and applying cold directly to trigger points or other tender areas. Ice helps numb the pain of a toothache or a sore finger, and it helps relieve muscle pain in the same way. A bag of frozen peas is ideal for this purpose as it moulds to the right shape, but remember to first wrap the bag in a cloth to protect the skin. A routine of ten minutes on, then ten minutes off, works best.

Cognitive dysfunction ('foggy brain')

Short-term memory loss, word mix-ups and difficulties with concentration are common problems in fibromyalgia. Cognitive dysfunction is usually attributed to the shortage of deep sleep and the fact that the individual's attention is often focused on trying to cope with the pain. The problem may also be intensified by fatigue.

Studies have failed to indicate any functional abnormalities in the memory and thought processes, but modern scanning techniques have shown that people with fibromyalgia have restricted blood flow to the parts of the brain controlling memory and concentration. The deep breathing and relaxation techniques outlined in Chapter 7 are excellent for improving the circulation to and through the brain. Hydrotherapy and stretching exercises aid circulation, too.

I suggest getting into the habit of writing things down, especially important dates and forthcoming events. Making lists may be tedious, but it is nice when you get to the shop and know exactly why you went there! Personally, I have found my lists of 'things to do' invaluable.

Morning stiffness

Morning stiffness – 'jelling phenomena' – is common in fibromyalgia. It generally occurs after the individual has spent maybe several hours lying in one position – overnight, for example, hence the name. In some people the condition is severe and may arise after sitting for a short time. The stiffness can take three or four hours to wear off and so may discourage a person affected from taking bus or car journeys or going to the cinema, theatre and so on.

Changing position regularly and moving around freely wherever possible does help. Walking around to avoid overnight stiffness is not practical, but getting straight into a hot bath or shower the next morning can minimize the discomfort. The employment of regular morning muscle-stretching exercises is helpful, too (see Chapter 5).

Irritable bladder

Many people with fibromyalgia have the feeling that their bladder is full most of the time. Urination may be painful and so a urinary infection may be suspected. Tests, however, usually show no evidence of infection. The problem is solely muscle irritation. If you find you need to urinate frequently, see your doctor. You may be referred to the urology department of your local hospital to learn exercises to strengthen your bladder muscles, which helps.

Dry eyes and mouth (sicca syndrome)

About a third of all people with fibromyalgia report dry eyes and dry mouth – 'sicca' means dry. Your eyes can burn and itch. If this is the case, you should inform your doctor. Eye drops, applied twice daily, will help to reduce the irritation and prevent reddening.

A dry mouth is likely to be caused by medication (antidepressant medications are notorious for this). It is therefore advisable to check the side effects of your prescribed drugs. Sucking boiled sweets or chewing gum is helpful, as is always having a glass of water nearby.

Restless arms and legs

Getting off to sleep is difficult enough for people with fibromyalgia. It can be distressing when, on top of that, your legs ache terribly, no matter how often you shift position. Then, when you have finally dropped off, worse is being snapped awake by jerking limbs or the fierce gripping pain of a leg cramp. Not pleasant!

Restless leg syndrome

Restless leg syndrome is not uncommon in fibromyalgia. It is characterized by an intense feeling of restlessness in the legs, particularly when you are lying in bed, trying to get to sleep. Cramps, especially in the calf muscles, are also associated with restless leg syndrome. Gentle movement, by walking around, can give temporary relief.

Nocturnal myoclonus

Sudden involuntary spasms in the arms and legs during sleep may also be experienced in fibromyalgia. This is known as nocturnal myoclonus – 'nocturnal' meaning night-time, 'myoclonus' meaning sudden contraction of the muscles. In severe cases, anti-spasmodic drugs may help. In mild to moderate cases, herbal remedies may prove beneficial (see Chapter 6).

Both of the above-mentioned sleep disorders can be frustrating for the person who has them and, when limbs start flying, not exactly pleasant for the person sharing the bed! In addition, they can severely interfere with sleep and the body's ability to rejuvenate the cells, recharging the batteries. As many experts regard these similar disorders as being caffeine-related, try cutting out caffeine products to see if it helps.

Numbness and tingling (paresthesia)

Paresthesia is the correct medical term for spontaneous burning, pricking, numbness and/or tingling – usually in the fingers and toes. When a doctor uses the term, it means that there is no obvious reason for the sensations, therefore further investigations need to be made.

When the underlying problem is fibromyalgia, it indicates that soft tissue problems (fibrotic muscles and so on) are interfering with the transmission of nerve messages. However, as with all the symptoms associated with fibromyalgia, they should never merely be assumed to be a part of the illness. Paresthesia may be a symptom of any one of several different conditions and should always be reported to your doctor.

Skin problems

Many people with fibromyalgia have sensitive skins. If the person is scratched so that a red mark appears, that mark will often linger for an unusually long time. This is particularly apparent in skin overlying the most painful regions, and is attributed to a hyperactive sympathetic nervous system. In other words, nerve messages are being inappropriately transmitted.

Irritations and rashes

Some people with fibromyalgia experience regular itching and rashes may develop. Hot baths, warm clothing and mild stress may make the problem worse. Rashes should be treated by the application of calamine lotion or hydrocortisone cream. There is, as yet, no known cause and treatment is not always successful.

Reynaud's phenomenon

Reynaud's phenomenon is an abnormal and exaggerated response to stimulation – cold or stress – that causes the blood vessels in the fingers and/or toes to narrow. The restricted blood flow then causes the affected areas to turn white or even bluish. The condition is almost always associated with disorders affecting the connective tissues – that is, the blood vessels, skin, muscles, tendons and joints – and so is occasionally found in individuals with fibromyalgia.

People who smoke can limit the attacks by giving up the habit. Smoking tends to narrow the blood vessels anyway and so will only exacerbate the condition. Reynaud's patients would be well advised to avoid drugs that cause the blood vessels to narrow further. The list includes some varieties of the oral contraceptive pill and some heart, blood and migraine medications. It is important that individuals with this condition remember to keep warm.

Temperomandibular joint dysfunction (jaw pain)

Facial pain affects about a quarter of the fibromyalgia population. For some it is part of the diffuse pain that characterizes the condition, but for others it comes from a malfunction of the temperomandibular joint (TMJ), which links the upper and lower jaws. Tense and fibrotic muscles and ligaments provoke pain in front of the ear on chewing and this is usually accompanied by a cracking or crunching sound. There may also be difficulty in opening the mouth. Other symptoms of TMJ dysfunction include headaches, facial numbness, dizziness and ringing in the ears.

The condition is commonly caused by traumatic impact, maybe as a result of a traffic accident, a fall, blow or even dental work. Dentists should be the first port of call where treatment is concerned. They may refer you to a dental specialist where a specially made splint worn over the lower teeth can greatly improve the situation.

Osteoporosis and fibromyalgia

The reduced activity levels common in people with fibromyalgia can lead to the early onset of osteoporosis, where the bones become brittle and more prone to fracturing. If left untreated, the condition can painlessly progress until a fracture occurs. Any bone can be fractured, but fractures of the spine and hip are of most concern due to their risk of serious consequences.

The condition is four times more common in women than in men, and a woman is more vulnerable if she is post-menopausal and experienced an early menopause. Unfortunately, I developed osteoporosis before I began to alter my diet, and it's not so easy to reverse. If you think you are at risk of this disease, ask your doctor to refer you to your local hospital for a bone density scan.

If you are diagnosed with osteoporosis, you will be prescribed medication to help your bones retain their calcium. Eating a calcium-rich diet can also prevent further calcium loss. Calcium-containing foods include dairy produce, dark green leafy vegetables (such as spinach, broccoli, spring cabbage and Brussels sprouts), shrimp, canned salmon and sardines, black strap molasses, calcium-fortified low-fat tofu and almonds. Some commercial foods, such as certain orange juices, cereals and yoghurts, are fortified with calcium and are highly recommended. It's advisable that, even if you have fibromyalgia and are *not* diagnosed with osteoporosis, you eat a diet that is rich in calcium and vitamin D (see below). Such a diet will help to prevent the future development of this bone-thinning disease. Drinking milk fortified with vitamin D is another good option – vitamin D is vital for enabling digested calcium to enter the bones.

You should also be aware that fresh fruits and vegetables contain essential minerals such as magnesium and potassium which help to reduce the elimination of calcium from the body. Magnesium-rich foods include dairy products, potatoes, beetroot, nuts, spinach, sole and halibut. Potassium-rich foods include bananas, oranges, prunes, potatoes, carrots, broccoli, avocados, lima beans, mushrooms, celery, alfalfa and cantaloupes. It's also worth noting that skimmed milk and non-fat dairy products provide as much calcium as full-fat milk and dairy products.

Recent research has shown that individuals who include more unsaturated fat in their diet are, on average, better able to absorb calcium than those on a low-fat diet. Therefore, this book advocates that 30 per cent of your food intake is fat in the form of polyunsaturated oils (canola, sunflower, olive and so on), as well as oily fish, avocados, nuts and seeds.

3

Medication

At last I had a diagnosis; at last I understood that my varied symptoms were all elements of one disease. 'So what can you do for me, doctor?' I asked. He pulled out his prescription pad and began to write ...

The need for chemical intervention

It is only natural that we look first to our doctors for help, and drugs are, almost without exception, the first course of action for the newly diagnosed. Only later do we look at other, more natural therapies that, unlike drugs, have neither side effects nor addictive qualities. However, as most drugs have an almost immediate effect and indisputedly go a long way towards suppressing the pain of fibromyalgia, they usually continue to play an important role in managing the condition, helping us live a more active, fulfilling life.

As people with fibromyalgia are often sensitive to medication, the benefits should always be weighed against the side effects. Commencing a course of medication on a very low dosage can markedly reduce the side effects. Remember that no one type of medication works for everyone. It is always wise to work closely with your doctor in order to find the drugs that are most suitable for you.

Painkillers (analgesics)

Painkillers are invaluable in fibromyalgia. Many doctors advise patients to take painkillers regularly, keeping the level in the blood more or less constant and thereby offering relief throughout the day. This works well for acute pain, such as that experienced during a flare-up but, as prolonged, high-dosage painkiller usage can lead to a reduction in its effectiveness (a situation whereby you need to take more and more to achieve the same result), addiction and eventually stomach, liver and/or kidney problems, it is not such a good idea for the long term.

In all but severe cases of fibromyalgia, the suppression of pain (barring that of flare-ups) can more safely be achieved by taking painkillers in lower quantities. Practising self-help pain management (see Chapter 7), a gentle exercise programme and improved posture (see Chapter 5) can go a long way towards alleviating pain without these negative effects. It is important, too, to learn to read your body. Painkillers taken before the pain intensifies are far more effective than painkillers taken when the pain is already severe.

Popular prescription painkillers include paracetamol, Tylex (30 mg codeine and 500 mg paracetamol), co-codamol and co-dydramol. In addition, an analgesic product by the name of Zydol (aka Tramadol) is now a popular choice with doctors. When prescribed to alternate with paracetamol-based analagesia in the treatment of moderate to severe pain, it is claimed to be as effective as morphine, but with fewer side effects. Zydol SR (slow release), on the other hand, offers the prospect of 24-hour pain control with only twice-daily doses. The severity of the pain should determine the dosage prescribed.

Over-the-counter painkillers

This category includes aspirin and paracetamol medications, each of which is capable of keeping mild to moderate pain at bay. Low-dosage codeine combined with paracetamol is also available over the counter. However, remember to inform your doctor of long-term over-the-counter drug usage. Over-the-counter painkillers are rarely powerful enough to deal with a pain crisis. It would be sensible, therefore, to have a few stronger prescription drugs to hand. Enteric-coated pills are easier on the stomach.

Many over-the-counter creams and gels have a warming, soothing effect. They can offer temporary relief from the pain of aching muscles or that of a muscle spasm. Used at bedtime, they can ease pain enough to promote sleep.

Narcotic analgesia

Fears of addiction have long prevented doctors from prescribing narcotic medications to chronic pain patients. However, many experts now claim that this important form of analgesia has been mistakenly withheld. We all know how addictive heroin and cocaine are, how the user can rapidly become a 'junkie'. Codeine and morphine are fellow narcotics, yet when used carefully to suppress chronic pain their addictive qualities are debatable. This is because codeine and morphine are unlikely to hit the 'pleasure zone' in the brain, and it is only when a drug hits the pleasure zone that the person craves more of the drug.

The fear of addiction was born after a 1998 study into the effect of morphine on terminally ill cancer patients. When escalating doses were required to achieve the same level of pain relief, doctors wrongly concluded that the drug was becoming less efficient. We now know that, in fact, the cancers had spread, causing increased pain, which required increasing amounts of the medication.

This error aside, because the body is adept at adjusting to changes within itself, long-term use of narcotic medication can actually cause the body to set up additional pain receptors and, for this reason, short-term use only is recommended. During attacks of acute pain, such as that experienced in a flare-up, narcotic medication can be very effective. It can not only relax a muscle spasm, it can also temporarily relieve anxiety and induce sleep – though not the deep sleep required in fibromyalgia – without fear of tolerance (where the patient needs to take escalating amounts to achieve the same effect). However, as with most medications, there are side effects. Narcotics can affect judgement, dexterity and short-term memory. They may even cause dizziness and nausea. All in all, when narcotics are treated with a lot of respect, they can be very useful.

Non-steroidal anti-inflammatory drugs (NSAIDs)

NSAIDs have both anaesthetic and anti-inflammatory qualities. They can be used to control the aches and pains of many disorders, particularly the most common forms of arthritis. However, because fibromyalgia is not a true inflammatory disorder, NSAIDs are only useful in flare-ups. Dizziness and nausea can arise in the short term, while prolonged usage can cause stomach and bowel irritation. Taking NSAIDs with meals can reduce or eliminate symptoms. As there are about a hundred medications in this category, your doctor may want to see how you respond to different ones. The only NSAID in tablet form available over the counter is ibuprofen.

Over-the-counter anti-inflammatory gels are rarely enough to minimize the pain of a muscle spasm or flare-up. Gels such as Feldene and Voltarol, massaged three times a day into painful areas, are known to be more useful, however. Consult your pharmacist or doctor about the best type of pain relief for you.

Antidepressants

Antidepressants are frequently the first line of treatment in fibro-myalgia – the primary objective being to boost serotonin levels. People with fibromyalgia, as we have seen, have low supplies of this important chemical.

In treating fibromyalgia, antidepressants are usually prescribed in lower doses than when used solely to treat depression. As explained in the previous chapter, depression in fibromyalgia is now seen as a reaction to the condition, rather than a cause of it.

Tricyclic antidepressants

Medications belonging to the tricylic group of antidepressants are most successful in reducing the pain of fibromyalgia. They work by increasing the concentration of certain chemicals (one of them being serotonin) that are necessary for nerve transmission in the brain and spinal cord. These chemicals are known to promote sleep, reduce pain levels and ease muscle tension. To prevent the feeling of a 'thick head' the following morning, tricyclic antidepressants are best taken in the evening rather than immediately before bedtime.

Tricyclic medications have several possible side effects. These include foggy brain, weight gain, constipation, dizziness, nausea, sweating, dry mouth and short-term memory problems. Taking this type of medication with food will lessen the chance of digestive problems.

There are many types of tricyclic antidepressants, all of which must be taken strictly as prescribed.

Anti-convulsants

The prescription drug pregabalin (brand name Lyrica) is now being recommended for the treatment of fibromyalgia. Pregabalin was previously used for controlling seizures, but recent studies have shown that it is of benefit in treating chronic pain conditions such as fibromyalgia, in a daily dosage of 300 to 600 mg. A person taking pregabalin will often notice improvements during the first week, but there may be side effects, including dizziness, drowsiness, dry mouth, blurred vision, constipation, larger appetite leading to weight gain, swelling of hands and feet, and problems with concentration and memory retention. Pregabalin may also possibly interact with certain other medications, such as antihistamines (usually taken to reduce allergic reaction) and medications for Parkinson's disease and diabetes.

If you have been prescribed pregabalin, build up the dosage very slowly, reporting any untoward or unacceptable side effects to your doctor. Should you miss taking a dose and it's nearly time for you to take the next dose, it's advisable to skip the missed dose. A study into the use of pregabalin in pregnancy is currently underway. If you have fibromyalgia and are pregnant, your doctor will advise you on whether or not pregabalin is a possible option.

Muscle relaxants

Muscle relaxants decrease muscle tension and are therefore useful for treating muscle spasms. They also help promote sleep. As long-term usage carries a high risk of tolerance and eventual dependency, it is not advisable to habitually use muscle relaxants to improve sleep. Also your doctor must be informed of any side effects. These may include dizziness, drowsiness, fatigue, flushing, headaches, nausea and nervousness.

When used to treat anxiety, medications in this category are very effective in the short term. It is important, however, to endeavour to discover the root cause of the problem – by seeing a trained counsellor, for example. When used to treat muscle tension, muscle relaxants are recommended for pain flare-ups only – and then never for longer than four weeks at a time. Listen very carefully to your doctor's advice before taking this type of medication.

Trigger-point injections

Usually lying at the centre of fibrotic bands of muscle, trigger points are areas of acute sensitivity that, when 'activated' (by overexertion, cold or a fall, for example), radiate pain into further areas. Anaesthetic injections – which should be administered only by pain specialists familiar with the fibromyalgia condition – work by breaking the cycle of pain within the tissues. The actual location of the injection – that is, whether or not it hits the most troublesome spot – determines the level of pain relief. Dry needling can be enough to break the pain cycle, but most specialists prefer to inject anaesthetic.

In most cases of fibromyalgia, the introduction of gentle exercise should then improve the quality of the tissues, gradually deactivating the trigger point and thereby reducing the radiated pain. The anaesthetic (lignocaine and its derivatives are most effective) acts for an average of three weeks, but continued benefit depends on whether or not the individual can successfully improve muscle tone during that time.

Epidural anaesthetics

Where trigger-point pain is severe and when anaesthetic injections fail to improve the situation, some pain specialists may consider administering an epidural anaesthetic. In this instance, anaesthetic is injected into the epidural space within the spinal column. This space lies between the vertebral canal and the dura mater (outer membrane) of the spinal cord. It is important that the procedure be carried out under X-ray guidance.

In cases of acute inflammation – that is, where bursitis is apparent (bursitis is inflammation of the fluid in the hollow that protects and surrounds a joint) – or when inflammation has occurred around the spinal cord, the anaesthetist may mix a steroidal medication with the anaesthetic. Obviously a high degree of precision is required for this procedure and you should ensure that your anaesthetist is well practised in this field.

Pain levels generally decline for longer periods than they do after trigger-point injections, giving the individual more time to improve the soft tissue situation.

Lignocaine infusions

Lignocaine infusions generally involve a seven-day stay in hospital. People must first be assessed to ensure that they are suitable for this type of pain relief. Blood tests and blood pressure readings are taken and the heart monitored by electrocardiogram (ECG). If all is well, you will be admitted about a week later.

During the first day in hospital, a fine tube (called a canula) is fitted and lignocaine anaesthetic medication administered by drip. You are wired to a heart monitor and your blood pressure is measured regularly. The daily infusion can take six to eight hours to complete and is administered over six days.

As with trigger-point injections and epidural anaesthetics, this treatment allows you a little 'breathing space' in which, with gentle exercise, the muscles can become stronger and more pliant. At present, most pain specialists are reluctant to offer this form of treatment on the NHS, although certain specialists in the West Midlands will take referrals from medical professionals in other areas of the UK.

Guaifenesin – does it work?

In recent years a medicine called guaifenesin, derived from the guaiac tree, has been put forward by some as a possible cure for fibromyalgia. However, there are plenty of others who assert that it is no more effective than a placebo (simple sugar pill). So what is the truth of the matter?

Guaifenesin was introduced as a medicine in the twentieth century and is a component of many over-the-counter cough and cold remedies, its function being to loosen phlegm and mucus in the lungs. An endocrinologist, Dr R. Paul St Armand, was the first to advocate its use in fibromyalgia after determining that the muscles in this condition become clogged by calcium phosphate build-up (a type of salt). He believes that guaifenesin prompts the kidneys to eliminate this and other unwanted stored matter from the body via urine and sweat. The urine is liable to become dark and pungent-smelling as a result. For years, the odour and colour-change was taken as a clear sign that something positive was happening and so seemed to confirm the efficacy of guaifenesin, as did the muscle aches, headaches, anal irritation, overwhelming fatigue and mild depression which arise during the therapy – however, these symptoms are difficult to cope with when you are already struggling with fibromyalgia. In fact, the therapy came with the warning, 'Not for wimps'.

In a book written in 2006, '*What Your Doctor May Not Tell You about Fibromyalgia: The Revolutionary Treatment That Can Reverse the Disease*, Dr St Armand asserts that guaifenesin therapy prompts a reversal of the fibromyalgia process, with increasingly longer cycles of symptom-free periods. He adds a strong warning that products containing salicylates should be avoided as they can interfere with guaifenesin function. Salicylate is a plant hormone, used in topical creams to ease aches and pains and reduce fever. It is also a key ingredient in make-up and many topical products for the treatment of acne, psoriasis, calluses, corns and warts. It is used in shampoos to treat dandruff, too. Interestingly, though, a one-year, placebo-controlled, double-blind study that was never published indicated that guaifenesin was no more effective than a placebo. Blood tests also showed that it could not possibly work as Dr St Armand believes (as shown below). When the chief author of the study, Dr Robert Bennett, was interviewed by the US Fibromyalgia Network, he stated that guaifenesin had been popular for so long because there were many Internet sites promoting it as a 'cure' for the condition – and what person with fibromyalgia could resist that?

The people who believe in the efficacy of guaifenesin claim that Dr Bennett's study was fatally flawed because patients may involuntarily have used salicylates, which would render the therapy ineffective. In the interview mentioned above, Dr Bennett gave several scientifically based reasons why guaifenesin therapy is 'grossly over-rated':

- In the study, both the serum and urinary levels of uric acid and calcium phosphate were all within the normal range and no increase in excretions was noted over time. Thus the postulated action of guaifenesin was not demonstrated.
- If some patients were using salicylates by some means, there would have been a significantly reduced urinary excretion and elevated serum level of uric acid. This was not observed.
- Dermatology consultants to Dr Bennett have explained that

patients would have to plaster their face with make-up several times a day to absorb enough salicylates to affect their urinary excretion of uric acid.

- In the early days of fibromyalgia, symptoms come and go on a cyclical basis, becoming more frequent and heightening in intensity as time goes by. Guaifenesin therapy is said to take the person back through those early days, except that the symptoms now show themselves in reverse order through increasingly shorter and less severe cycles. This claimed 'cycling of symptoms' was not observed in the study.

I have attempted here to present the facts of a contentious issue – so whether or not you try guaifenesin is entirely your choice. Plenty of people with fibromyalgia are still opting to use it in the belief that anything is worth a try. If it doesn't work, they say, there's no harm done.

4

Diet and the digestive system

I'd had trouble with my stomach for so long! Allergy testing suggested that yeast intolerance was my problem. Then some of my fibromyalgia friends also had tests. What a surprise! Most of them had yeast-related problems, too!

A dietary answer

Fibromyalgia is a disease in which the balance of the body is affected. There are problems within the immune system (our antibody protection against disease), the endocrine system (our hormone levels) and the central nervous system (our body's nerve signalling system located in the brain and spinal cord). These systems need to be supported by working from every angle possible to help the body back into balance. When, as a result, the bodily systems are once again networking properly, the errors will begin to correct themselves. The most vital area of support is improved nutrition for, among its many benefits, it is of enormous help to the body at the important cellular level.

The average diet in the West is composed of 60–70 per cent carbohydrates, 5–10 per cent protein and 25–45 per cent fat (most of it saturated, not unsaturated). These figures are based on percentages of calories, not grams. Eating such proportions of the different food groups invariably results in loss of muscle tone and shape, swings in energy and endurance, and slower mental focus (including concentration and short-term memory). As these problems are usually present anyway in fibromyalgia, it makes sense to say that improving your diet can greatly reduce the symptoms.

Studies of people with fibromyalgia have also shown that they lack the following:

- one of the important building blocks of life, i.e. the constituent that repairs muscle;

- an important transition fuel that helps to break down fat;
- a particular fuel source that results in reactive hypoglycaemia – a deficiency of glucose in the bloodstream.

The basic components of muscle and other soft tissues are proteins and minerals. Research has shown, though, that the average fibromyalgia sufferer eats a diet that is high in carbohydrates and low in protein – that was certainly me before I became interested in diet as a treatment. The human body is capable of repairing muscle and other soft tissues, but when it's deficient in protein, this restorative process will not take place. In fact, a diet low in protein will lead to increased pain.

So what can you actually eat? The diet recommended for the treatment of fibromyalgia comprises of 40 per cent *carbohydrate*, 30 per cent *protein* and 30 per cent *unsaturated fat*. These essential nutrients provide our bodies with vital energy and, as our bodies are in a constant state of regeneration, serve as fundamental building materials. You should also try to eat a moderately high amount of fibre. *Vitamins* and *minerals* are of almost equal importance and are discussed below. For more detail, see my book *The Fibromyalgia Healing Diet* (third edition, Sheldon Press 2014).

Recommendations for people with fibromyalgia

- *Eat three or four small meals a day, with snacks in between.* Try not to go more than two or three hours without eating.
- *Ensure you always have breakfast.*
- *Ensure your snacks are nutritious and readily available.* Good examples are raw fruit and vegetables, fruit and vegetable juices, dried fruit, unsalted nuts, seeds and rye crispbreads. People with fibromyalgia tend to have a lot of acid in their bodies. This can be combated by the alkalizing properties of fresh fruit and vegetables, which have a high vitamin and mineral content. Try not to eat too many tomatoes as they are highly acidic. Select locally grown, organic fruit and vegetables that are in season, and try to eat as fresh and as raw as possible. Try to make a variety of green salads and eat one every day.
- *Cook vegetables lightly.* When you have to cook your vegetables, use unsalted (or lightly salted) water and simmer for the

minimum length of time. Lightly steaming and stir-frying are healthy alternatives.

- *Eat legumes (peas and beans).* Legumes are cheap to buy and contain high amounts of protein, which is vital to the body for growth and maintenance. Protein also helps to relieve stiffness and pain. The soya bean is a complete protein, of which there are many derivatives including soya milk, tofu, tempeh and miso. Soya milk can be used as an alternative to cow's milk if you have an intolerance or allergy to this.
- *Include seeds.* Sunflower, sesame, hemp, flax and pumpkin seeds are very important for strengthening the body's systems. They can be eaten as they are as a snack, sprinkled onto salads and cereals, or used in baking.
- *Snack on nuts (unless you have a nut allergy, of course).* All nuts contain vital nutrients, but almonds, cashews, walnuts, Brazils and pecans perhaps offer the greatest array. Eat a wide assortment as snacks, with cereal and in baking.
- *Make your grains whole grains.* Whole grain and wholemeal flours provide us with the complex unrefined carbohydrates our bodies require – and again organic is best. Many types of grain are good for us, but wheat – our staple in the West – contains gluten and can be highly allergenic for some people. If you suspect you have a gluten allergy, ask your doctor if you can be properly tested. Although nutritious, wheat is acidic and not recommended in fibromyalgia. With the exception of wheat, aim to consume a variety of grains, including oats, rye, barley (generally available as pearl barley), corn, buckwheat, brown rice and mixed grains. Brown rice, millet, buckwheat and maize/corn are all gluten-free and invaluable to people with a gluten allergy or sensitivity.
- *Avoid salt, sugar and caffeine.*

A breakdown in the functions and processes within the digestive system is frequently found in fibromyalgia. In fact, many experts are now of the opinion that impaired digestion is actually one of the chief causes of the condition.

The factors leading to a digestive system breakdown may include stress and anxiety, eating too quickly, inadequate chewing, toxicity problems, the effects of antibiotic medications and a poor diet.

Abnormal gut microflora

Full health of the digestive system depends on an individual having ecologically 'balanced' gut microflora – the bacteria that help to break down foods. Friendly bacteria not only aid digestion, they also protect against invaders such as the parasitic yeast infection known as candida (*candida albicans*). The fact that many people with fibromyalgia suffer from chronic yeast infections is becoming more and more apparent.

Candidiasis is an infection caused by the candida fungus, usually of the *candida albicans* variety. In otherwise healthy people, candida infections are rarely serious, but when the immune system is depressed for some reason, candida can become a real problem. Certain medications – anti-inflammatory and immunosuppressive drugs, steroids and the Pill – can encourage candida to proliferate. People with nutritional deficiencies, people on high-sugar diets, diabetics and people who have suffered an illness that weakens the immune system – the obvious ones being AIDS and cancer – are also prone to developing candidiasis. Some evidence suggests that it can also be induced by coming off sleeping pills and tranquillizers after prolonged usage. Many experts also firmly believe that candidiasis can occur after a severe bout of 'holiday tummy' or after a gastric infection, particularly when someone has, in treating the upset or infection, taken a course of antibiotics.

Antibiotics can be very damaging to the gut microflora for they not only kill the micro-organisms that cause disease, but often kill much of the friendly bacteria, too.

Candida overgrowth (candidiasis)

Everyone has resident microflora in the gut that are capable of fermenting dietary sugars. It is only when the balance is upset and this type of microflora remains that fermentation actually takes place. When fermenting organisms are allowed to occupy a large area of the gut – which happens, for example, when antibiotics have killed much of the friendly bacteria – they multiply rapidly, producing alcohol and other toxins. Large overgrowths of candida can cause unsteadiness, clumsiness and slurred speech – drunken behaviour, in effect! The presence of this type of yeast infection can also interfere with the absorption of important nutrients into the bloodstream.

Candida does not arise as a result of *all* micro-organism fermentation, but it is a very common cause. However, when the candida is eliminated and balanced gut microflora restored, the individual is often relieved of many of the symptoms tied in with both fibromyalgia and irritable bowel syndrome (IBS).

The symptoms of candida overgrowth

Excessive amounts of intestinal candida can cause abdominal bloating and discomfort, alternating bouts of constipation and diarrhoea (or just diarrhoea), flatulence, indigestion, fatigue, depression, poor concentration, headaches (including migraine attacks), short-term memory problems, joint and muscle pains, and disturbed sleep – most of which are the primary symptoms of fibromyalgia!

When candida is eradicated and steps taken to ensure it does not recur, the symptoms of fibromyalgia can greatly recede. (There is no evidence, as yet, to suggest that they *totally* disappear.)

Gut fermentation

It is now known that when there is an overgrowth of candida, fermentation products are absorbed into the bloodstream. Tests have shown that blood alcohol levels rise significantly within an hour of the affected person eating sugar. When absorbed into the blood, these toxins (fermentation products) travel to the brain where ensuing adverse function can give rise to fatigue, depression, disturbed sleep, headaches and memory problems. As observed above, in some people, the candida overgrowth is so great they really can be mistaken for being drunk!

Yeast toxins

With the progression of the yeast infection (that is, the overgrowth of candida), toxins are released into the bowel, from whence they again are absorbed into the bloodstream, and this produces further symptoms. Some of these toxins have the effect of suppressing the immune system, some induce allergic reactions and others generate the production of antibodies that react against healthy tissues. In this instance, the ovaries may be attacked, causing premenstrual syndrome, irregular periods, reduced libido and so on, or the thyroid gland may be rendered inactive, with significant consequences.

A suppressed immune system, allergies and tissue damage are conditions often found in fibromyalgia. In fact, a suppressed immune system is considered, by some experts in the field, to be one of the major causes of the condition.

Yeast allergy

In addition, we now also know that the immune system can set up antibodies to the yeast organism itself. When this occurs, allergic reactions within the bowel can arise and allergic conditions, such as asthma and urticaria (an allergic skin rash) may develop. People affected will react against all foods containing yeast, as well as foods that advance yeast fermentation, such as sugar, alcohol and caffeine.

Permeability of the gut

In a healthy person, food is thoroughly digested before its products are absorbed into the bloodstream. Food will not slip through the bowel wall until the digestive enzymes have broken it down into minuscule units. Our immune systems do not recognize these units as foreign, simply because our bodies are made of the same basic building blocks as the foods we eat. However, when the gut wall is significantly damaged by fermentation products and allergic reactions to yeast overgrowth, food molecules are able to escape into the bloodstream before they have been properly digested.

Because these molecules are larger than usual – they are called macromolecules – the immune system recognizes them as foreign and so sets up antibodies to fight them. All healthy people absorb some of these macromolecules, but, because they are in relatively small amounts, the immune system can normally cope.

One theory about what happens next is that when vast amounts of these macromolecules are absorbed, the immune system, confused by the constant onslaught, begins to attack the body's own cells – the muscles, ligaments and so on – by mistake. It then sets up antibodies to foods other than yeasts and the body thus develops food intolerances.

By now you are probably wondering, how can you know for sure whether or not you have a yeast problem? In addition to the many symptoms outlined previously, a craving for sugar can be a good indication. Fermenting microbes thrive on sugar, therefore the individual affected can feel somewhat sugar deficient and, as a result, eat more sweet foods, which feed the yeast. Thus a vicious circle prevails. (Sugar cravings can also point to hypoglycaemia, a condition requiring urgent attention from your doctor. It is important, therefore, never to make assumptions about your health. Informing your doctor of all your health worries is essential.) Yeast problems are also indicated by recurrent bouts of oral, or, in women, vaginal, thrush.

You may wish to undergo 'allergy' testing, either as an in-patient at a special clinic, by asking your doctor to send off blood samples to a testing unit or by visiting designated premises (some health-food shops offer this test) for evaluation by a 'sensor' machine (although there is some doubt about the accuracy of the latter).

Note that, although you may present yourself for 'allergy' testing, the organization concerned will actually look for the foods to which you are 'sensitive' (see under 'Allergies', Chapter 2).

The yeasts in our environment

Yeasts are a group of microscopic fungi that exist in many different environments in nature. They may be present in our diet deliberately, as in baking and fermentation, or accidentally, as in overripe fruit and food that has been left lying around for too long. As sugar encourages the growth of yeast, removing all forms of sugar is recommended for individuals with a chronic yeast infection. Also, as the same individuals are often sensitive to yeast itself, all yeast products should be removed, too.

The elimination programme

Discovering whether or not you are sensitive to a particular type of food can be very difficult and each of the tests available can be criticized if you deliberately set out to do so. The only certain way to prove the case is via a food elimination programme, but to eliminate one food at a time, then to have to wait in order to assess your body's response, would take many months to do. For this reason, attending an 'allergy'-testing clinic is advisable. The results will at least point you in the right direction. Also, there are many 'allergy'-friendly foods and supplements available in healthfood shops and pharmacies.

Does food elimination have side effects?

Assuming that the foods eliminated were the right ones to start with, there is often an initial withdrawal reaction. Fatigue, headaches, twitching and irritability are normal symptoms, and can persist for up to 15 days. Drinking at least 2.8 litres (5 pints) of water a day helps to reduce such symptoms. It also aids detoxification, helping to flush any residual offending foods through the system.

A hypersensitive stage can then follow this period. If you have unwittingly eaten a food you are attempting to eliminate, the ensuing reaction can be severe, particularly when there is a true allergy. Dining out can be a problem, too. Ask the chef, not the waiter, if you are unsure about ingredients.

On a brighter note, a pleasing withdrawal symptom can be weight loss. The reason for this effect – assuming you are not starving yourself, which would be completely wrong and unnecessary – is that many people with food sensitivities have an unrecognized excess of fluid distributed throughout their bodies. When they begin to eliminate certain suspect foods, then start to feel better, the excess fluid quickly drains away.

It is important to note that a yeast-free diet will normally reduce the intake of calcium, protein, fibre, fat and B vitamins – all of which are obtained in a normal diet. However, this problem can be rectified by increasing consumption of cereals, vegetables, liver, fish – and by taking the 'allergy'-friendly B group of vitamins. All fruit should be thoroughly washed first, dried, then peeled and eaten immediately.

Elimination and reintroduction strategy

Should you wish to discover whether or not you have a yeast problem without going to the trouble and expense of allergy testing, try avoiding and keeping to the foods in Table 1 overleaf for a period of one month.

In addition, caffeine-containing drinks and foods (coffee, tea, chocolate, cola) should be avoided. These products induce a quick sugar-release that is not desirable where yeast has proliferated. If possible, try to avoid alcohol, too. It may be difficult when you are with other people. The thing to remember is not to be obsessive about it, just careful.

Make sure you are eating enough 'staple foods'. Cutting down too much can lead to nutritional deficiencies.

Table 1 Foods to avoid in identifying yeast intolerance

Foods to avoid		Alternatives
Cheese (including cottage and cream)	Spirits Monosodium glutamate (E621)	Perhaps the most difficult yeast food to replace is bread. However, healthfood
Ordinary bread	Mushrooms	shops now stock a sugar-,
Cakes	Soya sauce	yeast-, wheat-, egg- and
Pitta bread and buns	Tartare sauce	milk-free bread mix, to
Marmite		which you just add the flour
Stock cubes		of your choice. There are
Bovril	Watch out for 'leavening',	also soda bread, soda bread
Vinegar	'pickled', 'fermented' and	mixes, chapatis, matzos,
Pickles	'malt' on labels.	water biscuits, rye
Beer		crispbreads and rice cakes.
Wine	Chocolate containing	
Cider	sugar	For stock, use home-made,
Dried fruits		kept frozen, or vegetable
Yogurt	Removing all forms of	bouillon paste (available in
Salad dressings	sugar is recommended.	healthfood shops), broth
Ketchup		mix or soya cubes – all
Stuffing		made without yeast.
Tofu		

Table 2 Things to avoid if you are sensitive to fungi

Places that harbour water

Damp towels and clothing	Pet litter
Old peeling wallpaper and paste	Vaporizers
Leather goods	Potted plants
Paint that is peeling	Shower curtains
Overstuffed furniture	Rubbish bins
Foam rubber pillows	Vegetable bins
Hay and grain fields	Old mattresses
Poorly ventilated wardrobes	Leaky pipes and taps
Woodpiles	Refrigerator drip trays and rubber door gaskets
Roofs leaking into attics or behind walls	Compost piles or leaf piles
	Damp or flooded basements

Individuals who have an intolerance to yeast will also be sensitive to fungi – that is, moulds and mildew. The list in Table 2 gives examples of possible causes of asthma and chronic rhinitis.

Reintroducing excluded foods

Towards the end of the month, many of you should feel better than you have for a long time! The feeling of well-being can be so great you won't want to bother to reintroduce the foods you excluded.

However, for those who do wish to reintroduce those foods, the following procedure is suggested.

Day 1	In the morning, reintroduce a small amount of a food or drink previously eliminated (not a full-sized portion). Do the same later in the day. Record any symptoms.
Day 2	If you fail to experience symptoms, repeat the exercise. Once again, record any symptoms. If you get through the second day, this is really good news! Well done!
Days 3 and 4	Wait for two days before you can safely reintroduce this food into your diet on a fairly regular basis.
Thereafter	Repeat the above four-day reintroduction procedure with each food eliminated.

Any side effects should have occurred within four days. You may be disappointed, however, if your problem is not intolerance but true allergy. True allergies cause an immediate reaction – the immune system responds as if it is being invaded, thereby setting up antibodies to the offending food(s). Obviously you will need to continue to avoid this food.

If you do experience symptoms – for example, you develop a headache after reintroducing cheese – it would be better to leave cheese alone for at least six months before attempting to reintroduce it again. However, some foods will always cause an adverse reaction, so it would be wise to withdraw them from your diet altogether.

In the meantime, continue to eat sensibly. Try not to indulge too much in the foods that previously caused problems. Remember, if in doubt, leave it out!

Lack of vitamin and mineral absorption

Slow absorption may be the underlying problem in people who have multiple food sensitivities or true allergies. This usually means that essential vitamins and minerals are slow to be absorbed too and, consequently, the person will suffer deficiencies. This particularly applies to the water-soluble B group and C vitamins.

The individual will probably also have deficiencies in important minerals, such as magnesium, calcium, potassium, zinc and iron. In short, a person with multiple food sensitivities/allergies and so on should probably take multivitamin and multimineral supplements on a long-term basis. Your doctor's advice should be sought first, however.

Vitamins and minerals

When diet alone is not sufficient to replace vital sources of nourishment – as is often the case in fibromyalgia – supplementation can be the answer. As a result of a 1998 study, we know that people with fibromyalgia are frequently deficient in vitamins B3 and B6. When combined with magnesium and tryptophan – both of which have their sources in protein foods – these vitamins manufacture serotonin. As we have already learned, serotonin can reduce both pain and depression. It can also encourage much-needed sleep.

As many people with fibromyalgia are known to suffer magnesium deficiencies and as zinc and calcium also help induce sleep, it is recommended that fibromites take multimineral supplements. However, beware if you have a yeast infection. Selenium – also a mineral – is found in yeast. Some brands of multivitamins exclude selenium.

In short, you should probably be taking B complex vitamins, and to help your general nutritional state, vitamin C pills, in combination with selenium-free multiminerals.

Coenzyme Q10

Coenzyme Q10 (CoQ10 for short) is essentially a vitamin-like substance that plays an important role in the enzymatic process of producing energy in every cell of the body. CoQ10 is naturally present in a wide variety of foods, but primarily in organ meats, such as heart, liver and kidney. There is also a high concentration in beef, mackerel, sardines, peanuts and soy oil. Bodily tissues synthesize CoQ10 all the time, but many people are known to have a deficiency due, among other things, to inadequate diet or excessive utilization by the body.

As this enzyme is known to be concentrated in the muscle cells of the heart – the muscle that requires most energy production – several trials have taken place on patients with chronic heart disease. These trials established conclusively that heart function substantially improved and continued to do so for as long as CoQ10 was taken. Symptoms of fatigue as well as chest pain were considerably reduced, too. Because CoQ10 is believed to contribute to the control of cell growth, and because it undoubtedly energizes muscles, it is now being used by many people with fibromyalgia. It is hoped that funding for studies on CoQ10 and the fibromyalgia condition will be granted in the near future. Meanwhile, as this enzyme is remarkably side effect free, it is safe to take – although you must, first, see your doctor. By means of a blood test, your doctor will be able to determine your CoQ10 level. If it is low, the doctor can then monitor your progress as you take this important supplement.

Some people may require 100 mg of CoQ10 daily; others may need to take two or three times this amount to achieve the same blood level. CoQ10 is fat-soluble and so, although available in pressed tablet or capsule form, oil-based gelcaps are recommended. Its benefits are greater when chewed with a fat-containing food.

Vitamin D

Known as the 'forgotten vitamin', vitamin D aids calcium absorption and helps to form and maintain strong bones. It also works in concert with a number of other vitamins, minerals and hormones to promote bone mineralization. Without vitamin D, the bones can become thin, brittle or misshapen. Research also indicates that vitamin D helps to maintain a healthy immune system and assists in regulating cell growth and differentiation – the process that determines what a cell is to become.

A deficiency of vitamin D is now believed to be a major cause of unexplained muscle and bone pain. Indeed, in a study of 150 children and adults with unexplained musculo-skeletal pain, almost all were found to be severely deficient in this vitamin. A later study found that volunteers with pain were also vitamin D deficient, regardless of their ages. Cancers of the prostate, colon and breast are also linked with vitamin D deficiency, as are heart disease and auto-immune diseases such as rheumatoid arthritis and even type 1 diabetes.

One study, led by Dr Florian Wepner of the Orthopaedic Hospital, Vienna, Austria, found that vitamin D supplement helped relieve pain in people with fibromyalgia, especially those with low levels of calcifediol, a prehormone produced in the liver which is then converted to the active form of vitamin D.

It is possible to obtain vitamin D from foods and supplements, but this is not easy. A glass of fortified milk or orange juice contains about 100 IU of vitamin D, whereas a multivitamin typically holds about 400 IU. However, the recommended daily allowance (RDA) for fibromyalgia and unexplained pain is between 200 and 1,000 IU, depending on your age, sex and medical condition. Other sources of vitamin D are cod liver oil (1 tbsp equals 1,360 IU of vitamin D); salmon (75 g (3 oz) equals 425 IU of vitamin D); herring (75 g (3 oz) equals 765 IU of vitamin D); and canned sardines (75 g (3 oz) equals 255 IU of vitamin D).

However, we tend to obtain most of our vitamin D from exposure to sunlight. Therefore, people who seldom venture outdoors or always wear sunscreen are at risk of vitamin D deficiency. The message that all unprotected sun exposure is bad for you is too extreme. Indeed, experts now believe that a few minutes daily of unprotected sun exposure is important for health.

A fatty acid not often mentioned is omega 9, but if you suffer from inflammation it's just as important. It's often said that fibromyalgia is not an inflammatory condition, but in my worst years my neck and back were severely inflamed, and my wrists were so painful and swollen I was unable to move them and wore wrist braces all the time. It's clear, then, that fibromyalgia can cause inflammation, which can be reduced or eliminated by regular intake of omega 9 fatty acid. This acid is present in sesame and olive oil, avocados, peanuts, macadamia nuts, cashews, pistachios and pecans.

Other vitamin and mineral supplements

- *Vitamin C (ascorbic acid)* In fibromyalgia there is a shortfall of ascorbic acid. This vitamin is an excellent detoxifier and helps to reduce stress. Take up to 3,000 mg of vitamin C daily.
- *Vitamin B complex* As the B group of vitamins helps to reduce anxiety and stress, it is best to take a high potency B complex supplement twice daily.
- *Vitamin E* As vitamin E helps to improve sleep, alleviate fatigue,

boost healing and aid in the utilization of vitamin A by the body, you can take up to 400 IU daily.

- *Vitamin A (beta-carotene, the precursor to retinol)* This vitamin is necessary for the growth and repair of all bodily tissues. Take up to 10,000 IU per day.
- *NADH (nicotinamide adenine dinucleotide)* This coenzyme enables the body to increase adenine triphosphate (ATP), the fuel that provides the body with energy. Take 15–30 mg daily, depending upon the severity of your symptoms. The dosage should be reduced to 5 mg per day when your symptoms improve.
- *Calcium* This mineral works with magnesium to ensure proper muscle contraction/relaxations, and is important to good nervous system function. Take up to 1,000 mg daily.
- *Magnesium* As magnesium deficiency is universal in fibromyalgia, supplementation is highly recommended. This mineral is important for the absorption of many vitamins and minerals, and it aids the conversion of blood sugar to energy. Take 600–1,200 mg daily.
- *Manganese* This mineral plays a vital role in fibromyalgia, helping to create energy from glucose and aiding in the normalization of the central nervous system. Take up to 10 mg daily.
- *Zinc* Digestion, protein synthesis and good immune system function require plenty of zinc. Take up to 15 mg daily.
- *Potassium* This mineral works with sodium to regulate heart and muscle function. It also helps to ensure a correct acid–alkaline balance and normal transmission of nerve impulses. Take up to 5,000 mg daily.

Other useful supplements

- *Malic acid* This supplement plays a vital role in the operation of the 'malic acid shuttle service', which delivers important nutrients to the cells for conversion to energy. It is particularly effective when combined with magnesium. Some supplement manufacturers now offer *magnesium malate*, which combines the two. Take up to 200 mg daily.
- *Coenzyme Q10* As we have seen, this enzyme is important in fibromyalgia as it helps to increase mental and physical energy and alleviate pain and fatigue. It works by aiding the transfer of oxygen and energy between components of the cells and between the blood and the tissues. Take up to 100 mg daily.

- *Boron* This trace element is important to maintaining good muscular health. Because people with fibromyalgia may be inactive for long periods, it can also help to reduce calcium loss from the bones. Take up to 3 mg daily.
- *5-Hydroxytryptophan (5-HTP)* Because of its ability to increase serotonin levels, this phytonutrient (plant derivative) is useful in fibromyalgia for promoting sleep and reducing pain, anxiety and fatigue. The RDA for fibromyalgia is 100–500 mg daily, depending upon the severity of symptoms.

Vitamins A, C and E (known as the 'ACE' vitamins) together with CoQ10, zinc and manganese supplements work as fine antioxidants, reducing the oxidative stress of fibromyalgia and aiding the healing process. These substances may be purchased together in a single antioxidant supplement from certain health supplement manufacturers. Alternatively, the constituents may be bought separately, but generally at a higher price.

After one month of taking the above-mentioned vitamins and antioxidants, I suggest that you begin magnesium and malic acid supplementation. These nutrients work together to reduce pain, fatigue and low muscle stamina but, in the main, can only be bought separately. A multimineral supplement containing calcium, manganese, zinc, boron and magnesium should also be taken.

During the next month, you can start taking another of the recommended supplements, depending upon your choice. They all work in different ways to improve fibromyalgia. I appreciate that a fair amount of expenditure is called for – but, because of the many deficiencies in fibromyalgia, supplementation is important. Having said that, please remember that to take only one or two supplements is better than none at all. The antioxidant supplements are of prime importance, as is the magnesium–malic acid (magnesium malate) supplement. The dosages should be reduced to maintenance levels after eight to ten months.

Whether you go on to take any of the other supplements mentioned is entirely your choice, and perhaps dependent upon your finances. As some nutritional supplements interact with certain medications, and as they may adversely affect particular medical conditions, please consult your doctor before embarking upon a course.

Caffeine

You are probably aware that caffeine is addictive, but did you know that it has cocaine, morphine, strychnine, nicotine and atropine as close family members? More importantly, they are all nerve poisons. When it was first introduced to the UK, caffeine – from which the word 'coffee' is derived – was considered a severe health risk. However, coffee is now so socially acceptable that non-coffee drinkers are difficult to find. Consumed at regular intervals, products containing caffeine – including tea, chocolate, cocoa, and cola drinks – can give rise to chronic anxiety. This has as its symptoms mood changes, agitation, palpitations, hyperventilation, panic, insomnia, indigestion, headaches, nausea and weight loss. Unfortunately, individuals who display just a few of these symptoms often end up taking antidepressants, and in far higher doses than is normally necessary in treating fibromyalgia.

How much caffeine is 'safe'? Not much, although some people are far more caffeine-sensitive than others. Opinion varies regarding safety levels. Some experts consider that, in a day, four cups of coffee (or six cups of tea) are safe, while others believe the amount is nearer two cups of coffee (or three cups of tea). (Remember that a mug can contain twice as much as a cup, so that if you have mugs of tea or coffee, the safe amounts should be halved.) It can be deduced, therefore, that if you regularly drink in excess of four cups (two mugs) of coffee a day, you are overdosing on caffeine. Limiting your intake or, even better, cutting out caffeine completely, can make a terrific impact on the manifold symptoms of anxiety, which is one of the chief conditions associated with fibromyalgia.

However, as caffeine is very addictive, reducing your intake is far from easy. Withdrawal symptoms can take the form of splitting headaches, fatigue, depression, agitation, poor concentration and muscle pains. It's no wonder people can feel terrible until they have had their first dose of caffeine in the morning and can't seem to function properly without regular doses throughout the day! It also accounts for the headaches some people get when they sleep in on a Sunday morning.

Caffeine is 'washed out' of the system very quickly, however, so it's possible to minimize withdrawal symptoms by gradually reducing your intake over two or three weeks. Believe me, when it's totally removed from your system, you feel the difference!

5
Posture and exercise

I didn't know whether to laugh or cry when I was told that if I improved my posture and exercised regularly my pain would gradually lessen! Can't people understand that pain makes me slump and that exercise is simply agonizing?

Maintaining correct posture as we go about our daily activities is not easy. It demands that we are constantly aware of how we carry ourselves and that we always seek the easiest way to perform tasks. Our efforts in this area really are worthwhile, however, for repeated stress on muscles affected by fibromyalgia can cause pain levels to gradually rise.

Correct posture

How often were we told, 'sit up straight', 'don't round your shoulders', 'hold your head high' and 'don't slouch' when we were young? Slouching felt comfortable, though, and still feels easier than standing or sitting erect.

Slouching may still feel comfortable, but it stresses the muscles. Healthy people may, after years of slouching, suffer occasional discomfort in their lower backs; they may experience the odd twinge between their shoulder blades. People with fibromyalgia don't get off so lightly. Our reduced pain threshold means that poor posture can lead to intensely troublesome pain.

Unfortunately, maintaining proper posture is a real problem in fibromyalgia. Keeping our backs straight, our heads held high under the burden of severe pain is awfully hard work. Pain drags us down; it makes us want to hang our heads; it makes our bodies want to sag. Sadly, though, poor posture has the effect of encouraging further pain, which in turn causes our posture to deteriorate further. It is another of those vicious circles that keep appearing in relation to fibromyalgia. However, unless we learn to break out of these circles, our pain levels may continue to rise.

Breaking out of the vicious circle

Our backs consist of numerous internal and external muscles, all of which must be equally balanced in order to keep the lower back and pelvic regions correctly aligned. Activities that cause a shift in this alignment should be avoided – otherwise we risk incurring pain in our joints, muscles, ligaments and nerves.

Here are some basic postural recommendations that will help protect your body.

- When standing, ensure that your head sits over your shoulders (that it does not droop forward) and that your upper body is positioned directly over your feet (not with your hips forward so your spine forms an exaggerated 'S' shape).
- Try, at all times, to retain the slight hollow in the middle region of your back. When you are either still or performing an activity, your back should take on the form of an elongated 'S' (not the exaggerated 'S' mentioned above). Using a lumbar support will encourage the correct sitting posture.
- Stay relaxed. Maintaining correct posture does not mean tensing your muscles.
- Avoid slouching forwards or leaning backwards.
- Avoid twisting.
- Always have your work close to you.
- Warm up your muscles before performing any activity (see under 'Warm-up exercises' later in this chapter).
- Use the larger leg and arm muscles to perform tasks.
- Always seek the least physically stressful approach to an activity.
- Invest in energy-saving devices. Long-handled 'grabbers' are useful, as are 'shoppers' (on wheels), 'hands free' telephones, electric can openers, electric carving knives and food processors.
- Be as mobile as possible. Maintaining one position for an extended period aggravates the muscles. Keep stretching and shifting position.
- Alternate work with rest periods.
- As soon as your pain levels begin to rise, stop what you are doing and consider your options. These may include getting help, taking a break or cancelling the activity altogether. (Coping with your daily routine is discussed in greater detail in Chapter 7.)

Advice for specific activities

Housework

That ceaseless task that needs doing in every home is a real source of frustration to people with fibromyalgia. You battle with it at cost to your health until finally you think you have it licked. Before you've recovered enough to sit back and appreciate your efforts, you realize the whole lot needs doing again!

Before attempting housework of any kind, you should always consider the way you go about it. People with severe symptoms have little choice but to delegate most tasks to other family members. Encourage your children to earn their pocket money; explain to your partner that taking on the heavier work would be rewarded by seeing you a lot less incapacitated. If your partner has no time for housework or if you live alone, paying a cleaner to do the necessary tasks may be an acceptable alternative.

However, it may be time to consider living in less than perfect conditions, at least for the duration of a difficult spell. Although kitchen hygiene should never be neglected, a little dust and disorder elsewhere can do no harm. Try to make pleasurable activities your first priority – for what good comes of making your symptoms worse doing housework merely because you feel it is your duty or because you are worried that others will think badly of you for having a less than perfect home?

The following recommendations take account of both static and housework-oriented activities. Don't forget that, before undertaking any activity, you must first assess whether or not you are physically up to it. Try not to take chances and don't be afraid to delegate. Asking for help does not signify weakness on your part. Asking for help takes guts. It is an essential part of coping with your fibromyalgia (further advice on helping yourself with specific activities is given in Chapter 7). Learning to accept assistance is a sure sign that you are coming to terms with your fibromyalgia. In accepting the illness, you make a giant leap towards dealing with it successfully.

Sitting for long periods

There are times when you may need to sit for long periods – waiting to see the doctor/dentist, watching a play/film or at a family gathering, for example. Sitting, however, can put a lot of stress on the back and hips.

- If possible, sit in a chair that supports your entire back. (Chairs that look comfortable are not necessarily the most supportive.) Your chosen chair should have adequate lumbar support, armrests and seat you higher than a standard armchair. The added height makes it easier for you to stand up. Orthopaedic 'high chairs' can nowadays be purchased from larger furniture retailers, as well as from specialist outlets. If you are not in your own home, choose the best chair available – if necessary, politely asking another person to vacate the best seat, briefly explaining why you need a supportive chair.
- Ensure you always adopt the correct sitting posture. Your bottom should be tucked well into the back of the seat, your spine supported by the back of the chair. Your head should sit directly on top of your shoulders, so that your body carries its weight. Allowing your head to droop forward puts your neck muscles under terrific strain.
- Place a small cushion in the hollow of your back – around the level of your waist. This lumbar support encourages proper posture.
- Get up and walk around at regular intervals. If you are in someone else's home, explain that keeping as mobile as possible reduces your pain. If you are at the theatre, say, try to purchase seats at the end of a row. You will not then disturb people as you make regular trips to the loo, bar, confectionery kiosk and so on to give your back a break. If you are waiting to see your doctor, the dentist, rheumatologist or whomever, again, get up and walk around as often as you can. Peruse the noticeboards, take a couple of quick trips to the loo, stand looking out of the window a while. Don't worry about drawing attention to yourself; keeping your pain levels under control is of far more importance. If you are at home, remember not to sit for prolonged periods. When watching TV, use the breaks to have a wander – and 'lose' the remote control. You may prefer to lie on the sofa for a while to give your back a rest.
- If you are at home, place a hot water bottle at your back to relax the muscles. Requesting a hot water bottle from family and

friends will help your back stand up to the strain of sitting when you are visiting their homes.

Leaning over to read or write

As your head is the approximate weight of one of the heavier bowling balls – about 6 kilos (14 pounds) – it exerts enormous strain on your neck muscles. Leaning with your head forwards can, therefore, severely stress your neck and upper/middle back. Such positioning can also cause headaches. It is best to do the following:

- Invest (or ask your employer to invest) in a chair that supports your whole back. If you are unable to find such a chair at regular furniture outlets, Social Services should be able to supply you with details of a specialist chair manufacturer/retailer.
- Move the chair as close to the desk/table as possible to encourage proper posture.
- Ensure you are sitting straight, with your bottom pressed to the back of the chair. This should prevent you leaning forwards.
- Tuck in your chin as you look down – this will reduce neck strain.
- Bring your work closer to eye level. You may want to use a lap desk, drafting table or a secure box placed on top of your usual desk/table.
- Place frequently used work materials within easy reach.
- Tilt your head back every now and again to compensate for prolonged forward positioning.
- Take regular breaks. If you have a lot of paperwork to get through, keep getting up and walking around.
- Split the work into several short sessions. In the workplace, try to alternate 'looking down' tasks with duties where you can be more mobile.

Typing

Using a computer or typewriter can stress the back, neck, shoulders, arms, wrists and hands. Here are some guidelines to minimize this:

- Follow the above recommendations for sitting at a desk/table.
- Use the computer's tilting feature to find the best position. When you are seated, the top line of the screen should be no higher than eye level. Positioning the screen too high will cause unnecessary neck strain.

- Ensure that the screen is directly opposite you. Looking to one side for prolonged periods can severely strain the neck muscles.
- If possible, adjust the height of your chair or work surface so your forearms are parallel with the floor and your wrists are straight. Sitting at a low work surface encourages poor posture.
- Invest in (or ask your employer for) a foot rest. This will reduce the pressure on your lower back.
- The mouse and other input devices should be positioned so that your arms and hands are in a relaxed and natural position.
- Position the keyboard directly in front of you. This makes it possible to type with your shoulders and arms relaxed.
- If you use a document holder, position it at the same level as the computer screen.
- Position the mouse at the same level as the keyboard.
- When typing, keep your wrists in a straight and natural position.
- Keep your elbows in a relaxed position by your sides.
- Use the minimum force required to push down the keys.
- Purchase an ergonomic wrist rest for your keyboard. This should help to reduce (or prevent) tendon pain – similar to that of repetitive strain injury (RSI) – in your hands and wrists.
- Purchase (or ask your employer for) an ergonomic keyboard.
- Flex your hands and wrists every ten minutes.
- If required, use a wrist splint to minimize wrist mobility.
- If using a conventional mouse, move it with your whole arm.
- If possible, use a computer mouse containing a trackball. This will limit wrist movement.
- Using an ergonomically 'moulded' mouse will support your hand and wrist.
- Take regular breaks. You will find that frequent, short breaks are far more beneficial than fewer, longer breaks.
- Stand and take a few minutes to stretch your muscles between breaks.
- Give yourself a time limit. When it is up, break off until later. (Should your pain levels begin to rise before your time is up, finish what you are doing immediately.)

Reaching up to perform a task

Performing an activity while reaching upwards – say, taking crockery down from a high shelf, replacing a light bulb, hanging curtains – can put your back, shoulders and arms under enormous strain. It is best to:

- stand on a small stool (one you know to be stable) so you don't have to stretch);
- use a long-handled implement for inaccessible cleaning jobs;
- take regular breaks to minimize strain;
- store items in general use – such as groceries, pans, crockery and so on – in more accessible cupboards.

Washing-up, preparing vegetables and so on

Leaning over kitchen worksurfaces for prolonged periods can stress the neck and back. It is best to:

- move as close to the worksurface as possible to encourage proper posture;
- stand tall, making sure to tilt your head and tuck in your chin;
- place a wooden box on the worksurface to bring the work closer (maybe someone keen on DIY could make you one);
- take regular breaks;
- stop altogether as soon as you feel your normal pain levels begin to rise.

Carrying shopping and so on

Carrying heavy shopping and other items in your hands, with your arms extended, exerts great strain on your shoulders, arms and back. It is best to:

- park as close as possible to the supermarket or shop;
- take someone with you so you can share the load;
- limit the amount you carry at one time – two journeys carrying less are better than one journey involving carrying lots of bags or boxes;
- carry items close to your body, wrapping your arms around your packages, as carrying loads close to the body disperses the strain;
- ensure the load is balanced;
- use a shopping trolley on wheels, or make use of the facility

some of the big supermarkets offer of a shop assistant taking the shopping to your car for you (alternatively, you could try using Internet or phone shopping services that do the shopping and then deliver it to you, although these are not yet available throughout the country).

Lifting a bulky object off the floor

Bending forward to lift something like a full laundry basket can strain the whole back – the lower back being particularly vulnerable. When lifting, you should be careful to ensure your legs, rather than your back, take the strain. The golden rule is, therefore, LNB – which stands for 'legs, not back'. A reminder, too, that you must assess, first of all, whether or not you are really up to lifting. If you choose to go ahead, it is best to:

- plant your feet about 30 cm (12 in) or so apart – a wide base helps maintain correct alignment;
- keeping your back straight, bend your knees until you are resting on your haunches, then place your arms around the object;
- push upwards with your legs in order to raise it from the ground;
- if possible, break the load into smaller portions – where laundry is concerned, it is safer to lift a few items at a time, carrying them close to your body (perhaps over your arm if the items are dry) to the washing machine, tumble drier or clothes airer;
- if the object is larger than a laundry basket, get someone to help.

Carrying a bulky object

Because oxygen is not readily converted into energy in fibromyalgia, carrying can severely stress the hands, wrists, arms, shoulders, neck and back. It is best to:

- keep the object close to your body as you walk, ensuring your grip on it is firm;
- maintain an upright posture, again ensuring that your legs – not your back – take the strain (LNB);
- rest the object on an available surface – a table or worksurface – to give your muscles a break during the carrying time.

Setting down a bulky object

Lowering a bulky object down on to the floor stresses the lower back in particular. It is best to:

- plant your feet about 30 cm (12 in) apart;
- keeping your back straight, bend your knees, letting your legs take the strain as you lower the object to the floor (LNB once more);
- if transporting laundry, for example, from the kitchen to the outside washing line, setting the basket on a nearby patio table, garden bench or a broad-topped wall will save you the strain of lowering it to the ground.

Picking something light up off the floor

Most people tend to arch right over to pick a piece of fluff, for example, off the carpet. This can put enormous strain on the back – the lower back in particular. It is best to:

- keep your back straight, bending your knees until you are able to reach the object;
- use your thigh muscles to propel you upright again (LNB);
- if your leg muscles are too weak/painful to do the above, use a long-handled 'grabber'.

Putting a casserole in an oven

Bending forward at the waist while carrying heavy things with your arms outstretched puts a great deal of stress on your back. Holding something heavy away from your body increases that strain. It also stresses the tissues of the hands, wrists, arms, shoulders and neck. If your oven is below worktop level, it is best to:

- stand close to the open oven, holding the casserole dish in both hands;
- keeping the dish close to your body, drop down on to your haunches and slip the dish into the oven (LNB);
- push yourself upright again with your thigh muscles (simply reverse the procedure to remove the casserole from the oven).

Putting laundry into the washing machine

Bending to push clothes and so on into the washing machine can stress your back and shoulders. It is best to:

- lower yourself into a kneeling position, keeping your back straight;
- push only a small amount of washing in at a time – several repetitions are better than trying to thrust in a great bundle at once (reverse the procedure to remove the washing).

Lying in bed all night

Lying down for long periods can make you feel stiff and sore. In particular, lying on your back puts a lot of pressure on your back and hips. It is best to:

- place a pillow beneath your knees to take the strain off your lower back;
- use no more than one pillow to support your head and neck – moulded cervical pillows keep the head correctly aligned during sleep;
- turn on to your side to relieve the pressure on your back and place a pillow between your knees to take the strain off your hips;
- don't sleep on your stomach;
- use a reasonably firm mattress – mattresses that sag will only contribute negatively to your problems.

Driving a car

Driving can stress virtually every muscle in the body. It is important to assess whether or not you are up to driving in the first place. If you believe you are, it is best to:

- adjust the seat so it is as near the steering column as is comfortable;
- make sure the back of the seat is adjusted correctly – it should be neither too upright, nor reclined too far;
- don't slouch or allow your head to drop forward;
- wear an inflatable neck support;
- use a lumbar support (a cushion in the small of your back will do);

- make sure your car has a headrest and adjust it to suit your height – in the unlucky event of a collision, the headrest can minimize the severity of whiplash injury;
- when driving, armrests can reduce stress on the arms, shoulders and upper back – they can also help support the upper back when you travel as a passenger;
- use your wing mirrors when reversing rather than turn round unnecessarily;
- when changing your car, pick one with very light steering;
- when buying a new car, choose one with an automatic gearbox – this will eliminate the need to depress the clutch and shift the gear lever;
- electric windows, wing mirrors, sunroof and so on are easier to manage than their manually controlled counterparts;
- make regular breaks in a long journey to walk around and stretch your muscles;
- share the driving with someone else.

When travelling as a passenger, follow the relevant steps above to ensure that you are sitting properly as this helps to minimize the stresses on your body.

Rising from a chair

Jerking your upper body forwards in order to get out of your seat can stress the muscles of your entire back. It is best to:

- move your bottom to the edge of the seat;
- place one foot as far backwards as possible;
- use the armrests to help propel you upwards, making sure you don't lean forwards as you stand.

Getting out of bed

Twisting your body to get out of bed (or off the sofa) can put the back and hips under a lot of strain. It is best to:

- roll on to your side, bending your knees so they hang slightly over the edge of the bed;
- move your feet outwards and over the edge of the bed;
- place the palm of your uppermost arm on the bed at the level of your waist and, as you push your body upwards, swing your legs

down until they touch the floor – this should smoothly propel you into a sitting position.

Exercise

For years we have known that inadequate exercise can aggravate fibromyalgia. Surprisingly, it is now widely believed that it can also contribute to the onset of the condition. Many people who develop fibromyalgia following a physical trauma report that their activity levels were, probably for reasons of self-protection, reduced significantly following the initial trauma. Now that we are aware of this factor, it is hoped that doctors will, at some point in the future, be able to slow down or even prevent the illness. This would be done by monitoring physical trauma patients more thoroughly – particularly those suffering whiplash injuries. Ensuring they are taught correct posture and that they are set a home exercise regime should, hopefully, be a part of their post-trauma treatment.

Adopting a physical exercise programme has long been hailed as being beneficial for people with fibromyalgia. When it is persevered with in conjunction with other treatment regimes – improved diet, antidepressant medication, self-talk and so on – the improvements can be profound. Think about and choose your forms of exercise with care, making sure you do not decide on something that will be difficult to keep up because, for example, a class takes place some distance away. Be flexible, too, as variety keeps it interesting and enjoyable. Ensure there is something you can do whether you are well or not feeling so good.

Why exercise?

The majority of people with fibromyalgia have made efforts to exercise, but are put off further attempts by a subsequent rise in their pain levels. After all, the knowledge that physical activity will, in all probability, generate further pain is far from encouraging. Also, bad experiences of exercise can not only decrease motivation, they can also induce exercise phobias.

It is a sad fact that when we first start an exercise programme, the pain is likely to temporarily increase. This occurs because our muscles are tight and out of condition. However, unfortunately, the only way to stretch and strengthen the muscles is to exercise them. Without exercise our bodies are liable to become increasingly painful – prolonged inactivity, ultimately, causing our muscles to waste. However, as explained below, any activity or exercise producing more than a slight increase in pain should immediately be curtailed.

An individually tailored regime

The severity of the symptoms related to fibromyalgia varies considerably from person to person. The pain and fatigue also affects people differently. It is advisable, therefore, that each person develops a personalized routine. This routine should depend largely on which activities you are most able to do without provoking more pain, as well as on those you enjoy the most.

As you read through the exercise possibilities – given below in order of progression – make a note of the ones you think you may be able to do. Remember that even if only warm-ups may be within your scope at the outset, you should be able to expand your routine as your muscles gain in flexibility and strength.

Take care not to overdo it

Unfortunately, there are still some people who believe that people with fibromyalgia simply need to 'push themselves' in order to improve their condition. If only it was that simple … Your doctor or physiotherapist may even believe that regular vigorous exercise is the only way to increase depleted levels of certain growth hormones, which are essential for the repair and regeneration of the tissues. However, recent research has found that exercise does not increase the production of growth hormones in fibromyalgia. In fact, vigorous exercise is known to cause microscopic tears in the muscle tissues (microtraumas). In healthy people such tears may promote slight stiffness, but people with fibromyalgia – a disease of pain amplification – often experience the tears as severe pain.

Don't let anyone tell you that although your pain may feel severe, your muscles are not badly affected. We now have evidence that strongly indicates that prolonged muscle pain causes pain-transmitting chemicals to continue to build, which, in turn, causes pain levels to continue to rise. The higher the levels of pain, the more stress and tension is induced, with the usual knock-on effect on the tissues (see Chapter 1 for more details regarding pain amplification). Because of this, any activity should be undertaken with extreme care.

It makes sense to say, then, that in attempting to formulate an exercise routine, it is important that people with fibromyalgia refrain from pushing themselves beyond their known limits. Although a little added discomfort should be expected, it should not exceed the stage where it will not 'rest off' during the remainder of the day and overnight.

After warming up, perform one or two of the easier stretching exercises. If your stiffness, fatigue and pain levels remain higher than normal the following day, either you did not allow sufficient resting time for your body to recover or your chosen exercise was, in fact, overambitious. Allow your body a further two or three days to recover, then recommence your routine with a more basic exercise, and make sure you get enough rest afterwards. As you finish your exercise routine, you should feel as if you could have done more. Bear in mind that you may be able to achieve the dropped exercise when your muscles are stronger.

It is recommended that, for several days, you think carefully about all the exercises described. You may perhaps want to rank the exercises, placing an asterisk against those you think you can attempt, then two asterisks beside the easier of them, starting your routine with these. You may decide to aim to do 15 minutes' exercise a day, but, to be safe, you should spend only 2 or 3 minutes exercising at the outset. On the other hand, your objective may be to exercise for an hour. This is not advisable. It is far safer to break exercise sessions into two parts, completing a second session later in the day if you still feel up to it.

Activities/movements to avoid

A contracted muscle will shorten and appear larger – such as a contracted biceps muscle, which bulges when the elbow is bent. Working muscles – those being exercised – move by means of 'concentric contraction'. Like a working biceps muscle, they, too, shorten and may appear larger. 'Eccentric' contraction occurs when a muscle is shortened, but is being forced to lengthen. This happens when you are lifting something as well as stretching – for example, when stretching to place a heavy pan on a high shelf. The biceps muscle contracts because the pan is heavy, yet you have to extend your arm to reach the shelf. Forcing muscles to stretch while they work can cause small tears in the muscle tissues (microtraumas), which take time to heal. As we saw earlier, microtraumas can be very painful.

Identifying and eliminating eccentric muscle movement is an important part of reducing the pain of fibromyalgia. It can be learned, so long as you try to focus on all that you do. Vacuuming is a typical example of eccentric movement. You contract your muscles to grip the handle of the cleaner, yet at the same time you push it backwards and forwards. For this reason, filling a dishwasher is also hard on the muscles, as are putting dishes away, hanging out washing, gardening, hammering, sawing and so on.

You may be surprised to learn that swimming, too, is not recommended for people with fibromyalgia. Although the water supports the body, the arm movements required for most strokes involve this eccentric contraction. Water exercises can be a beneficial alternative, however, and you may want to join an aqua-aerobics class (see under 'Aerobic exercise' later in this chapter).

Warm-up exercises

Many muscle groups are permanently tight and prone to being painful. If you try to move them beyond a certain point, they may resist and forcing them only makes them more painful. It is essential, therefore, that warm-up exercises are performed at the start of your routine. Warm-ups should include mobility exercises for your joints, simple pulse-raising activities for your heart and lungs and short, static stretches for your muscles.

Although I have described the warm-up exercises recommended for people with fibromyalgia generally, the ones you choose should depend largely on your own limitations. For example, a person with severe symptoms would be advised to formulate a very gentle programme. One or two repetitions of several exercises are generally better than several repetitions of only one or two exercises. A person with milder symptoms can devise a more challenging programme, lasting maybe 15 to 30 minutes. In the latter instance, warm-ups should last up to ten minutes and be slightly more energetic than in the former case.

Note: Never skip warm-ups in favour of more vigorous exercise.

Mobility exercises

These exercises should be smooth and continuous. It is important, too, that you keep your body relaxed. Exercising when tense can cause more harm than good. Remember to keep your back straight, your bottom tucked in and your stomach flattened as you perform your routine. You should stand with your legs slightly apart.

Shoulders

Letting your arms hang loose, slowly circle your shoulders backwards. Repeat the exercise two to ten times, depending on your condition. Now slowly circle your shoulders forwards and repeat between two and ten times, as appropriate.

Neck

1 Making sure you are standing straight, slowly turn your head to the left – as far as it will comfortably go – then hold for a count of two. Return to the centre and repeat the exercise between two and ten times. Now turn your head to the right, holding for a count of two before returning to centre. Repeat between two and ten times.
2 Tucking in your chin, tilt your head down and hold for a count of two. Repeat between two and ten times. Again tucking in your chin, tilt your head upwards, but not so far that it virtually sits on your shoulders, and hold for a count of two. Repeat between two and ten times.

Spine

1 Placing your hands on your hips to help support your lower back, slowly tilt your upper body to the left and hold for a count of two. Return to the centre, then repeat between two and ten times. Now tilt to the right and return to the centre. Repeat between two and ten times (see Figure 3).
2 Keeping your lower back static,

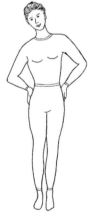

Figure 3 Spine mobility exercise

gently, in a flowing rather than fast movement, swing your arms and upper body to the left as far as it will comfortably go, then return to the centre. Repeat between two and ten times. Now swing your arms and upper body to the right and return to the centre. Repeat between two and ten times.

Hips and knees

With your body upright, move your hips by lifting your left knee upwards, as far as is comfortable. Hold for a count of two, then lower. Now raise your right knee and hold for a count of two. Repeat between two and ten times (see Figure 4).

Ankles

With your supporting leg slightly bent, place your left heel on the floor in front of you. Lift up your left foot and then place your left

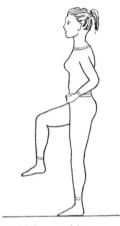

Figure 4 Hips and knees mobility exercise

toes on the floor. Repeat between two and ten times. Now duplicate the exercise and number of repetitions with the right foot (see Figures 5(a) and (b)).

Pulse-raising activities

Still part of your warm-up routine, pulse-raising activities must be gentle and should build up gradually. Their purpose is to help warm your muscles in preparation for stretching. Walking around the room for two to four minutes, followed, if possible, by walking once up and down the stairs is ideal.

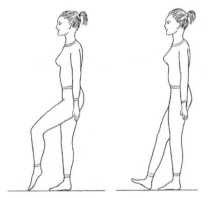

Figures 5(a) and (b) Ankle mobility exercises

Stretching exercises

The muscles, already becoming warm and flexible, relax further when short stretches follow mobility and pulse-raising activities. Stretches prepare them for the more challenging movements that, hopefully, follow. These exercises have been devised with the help of the Health Development Agency.

Again, it is up to you to decide which you think you are capable of performing. On days when you feel a little more delicate than usual, carrying out a few stretching exercises should help to relax the muscles.

Calves

1 Stand with your arms out-stretched, your palms against a wall. Keeping your left foot on the floor, bend your left knee and stretch your right leg out behind you. Press the heel of your right foot into the floor until you feel a gentle stretch in your leg muscles. Now change over legs. Repeat between two and ten times (see Figure 6).

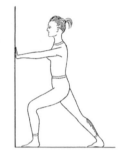

Figure 6 Stretching exercise for the calves

2 Standing with your feet slightly apart, raise both heels off the floor so that you are on your toes. Repeat between two and ten times. As your calf muscles strengthen, you should be able to stay on your toes for longer periods of time. This exercise also helps your balance.

Fronts of the thighs

Using a chair or wall for support, stand with your left leg in front of your right, both knees bent, your right heel off the floor. Tuck in your bottom, and move your hips forwards

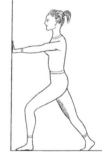

Figure 7 Stretching exercise for the fronts of the thighs

until you feel a gentle stretch in the front of your right thigh. Now change over legs. Repeat between two and ten times (see Figure 7).

Backs of the thighs

Stand with your legs slightly bent, your left leg about 20 cm (8 in) in front of your right leg. Keeping your back straight, place both hands on your hips and lean forwards a little. Now straighten your left leg, tilting your bottom back and until you feel a gentle stretch in the back of your left thigh. Now change over legs. Repeat between two and ten times (see Figure 8).

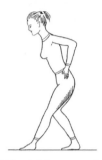

Figure 8 Stretching exercise for the backs of the thighs

Inner thigh

Spreading your legs slightly, your hips facing forwards and your back straight, bend your left leg and, keeping the right leg straight, move it slowly sideways until you feel a gentle stretch along your inner thigh. Gently move to the right, bending your right leg as you straighten the left (see Figure 9).

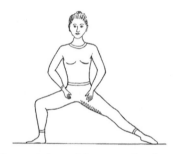

Figure 9 Stretching exercise for the inner thigh

Chest

Keeping your back straight, your knees slightly bent and your pelvis tucked under, place your arms as far behind your lower back as you can and your hands gently on your lower back. Now move your shoul-

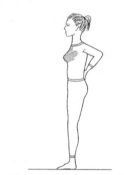

Figure 10 Stretching exercise for the chest

ders and elbows back until you feel a gentle stretch in your chest (see Figure 10).

Back of the upper arms

With your knees slightly bent, your back straight and your pelvis tucked under, raise your left arm and bend it so that your hand drops behind your neck and upper back. Using your right hand, apply slight pressure backwards and downwards on your left elbow, until you feel a gentle stretch (see Figure 11).

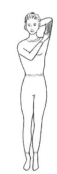

Figure 11 Stretching exercise for the back of the upper arms

Note: Most people with fibromyalgia have some muscle groups that are far tighter than others – often the neck and shoulders. To reduce the gradual build-up of pain in these areas, you will benefit from gently stretching the relevant muscle groups at intervals throughout the day.

Strengthening exercises

Not all people with fibromyalgia can tolerate strengthening exercises, so use caution, beginning with one or two repetitions of your chosen exercises. Although the movements may seem easy at the time, the real test is how you feel the next morning.

The following exercises help condition the muscles required for pushing, pulling and lifting. They will also help increase your stamina. Remember to incorporate small pauses between repetitions, focus on staying relaxed and don't forget to breathe as you exercise.

Thighs

1 The large muscles running along the tops of your thighs (the quadriceps) quickly become weak when you are inactive. Strengthening exercises will help you walk, climb stairs and get into and out of chairs more easily. Lean back against a wall, your feet 30 cm (12 in) away from the base of the wall. Adopting

correct posture, slowly squat down, keeping your heels on the ground. (Don't go too far down at first.) Now slowly straighten your legs again. Repeat between two and ten times, lowering your-self further as, over time, your muscles strengthen.

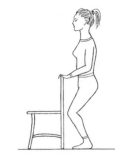

Figure 12 Strengthening exercise for the thighs

2 Holding on to a sturdy chair and keeping your back 'tall', bend and then slowly straighten both legs, keeping your heels on the floor. Repeat the exercise between two and ten times (see Figure 12).

3 Sit in a chair and push your knees together, tightening your thigh muscles as you do so. Hold for a few seconds. Repeat between two and ten times.

Upper back

Lie face down on the floor, hands by your side, not on the floor, and keeping your legs straight and tightening your stomach and back muscles, gently raise your head and shoulders. Hold for a count of two, then lower. Repeat between two and ten times (see Figure 13).

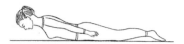

Figure 13 Strengthening exercise for the upper back

Lower back

Lie on your back, using a small rolled cloth or towel to support your neck, then lift your knees, keeping your feet on the floor. Lift first your left leg gently

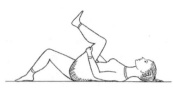

Figure 14 Strengthening exercise for the lower back

behind the knee, pulling it towards your chest until you feel a gentle pull in your bottom and lower back. Repeat with the right leg. Now pull both legs up together. Repeat each exercise between two and ten times (see Figure 14).

Abdomen

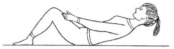

Figure 15 Strengthening exercise for the abdomen

1 The abdominal muscles commonly become very weak in people with fibromyalgia. However, the stronger they are, the more they support your back. Lie on your back, using a small rolled cloth or towel to support your neck. Lift your knees and place your feet flat on the floor. Now tighten your abdominal muscles, tuck your chin in a little towards your chest and raise your head and shoulders, reaching with your arms towards your knees. Remember to keep your lower back pressed down on the floor (see Figure 15).

2 If you are not up to doing sit-ups, the following exercise is just as effective. Lie on your back, using a small rolled cloth or towel to support your neck. Pull in your stomach muscles and try to flatten your spine against the floor. Hold for a count of two, then release. Repeat between two and ten times.

Arms

Place your left hand on your chest and press for a few seconds. Do the same with your right arm. Repeat between two and ten times.

Push-ups

Stand with your hands flat against a wall, your body straight. Carefully lower your body towards the wall, then slowly push away. Repeat two to ten times. At first, stand quite near the wall, then try moving further away as you become stronger (see Figures 16(a) and (b)).

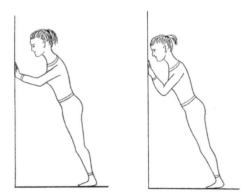

Figures 16(a) and (b) Push-ups

Using small weights

People with milder symptoms may now be able to increase their strength by using small weights. The type that fasten with Velcro around the wrists and ankles are recommended. Weights of 225 g (8 oz) each slip into small pockets sewn into the band. Such weights are available from most sports shops. Start by using one weight only.

1 With the weights around your wrists, stand with your feet slightly apart. Making sure that only your upper body moves, turn carefully to the left, swinging both arms gently as you move. Repeat two or three times. Now perform the same exercise and number of repetitions, but this time swing your body and arms to the right. Ensure the movements are steady and fluid, not too fast.
2 Keeping your left elbow close to your waist, slowly raise your left forearm so it almost touches your shoulder. Lower the forearm until it is at right angles with your upper arm, then slowly raise it again. Now repeat the exercise with your right arm, again ensuring your movements are steady and continuous.
3 Bending your left arm, bringing your hand up until your wrist is level with your shoulder, reach your hand upwards until your elbow is level with your shoulder. Bring it straight back down to the original position. Repeat once more, then do the same with your right arm.

As you gain in strength and flexibility you may be able, first of all, to increase the number of repetitions you do and, second, to add to the weight you lift. If your pain levels are higher than normal the next day, however, I recommend that you postpone these exercises until you feel stronger.

Walking with weights

Using the Velcro weight bands described above as you walk around the house, up and down the stairs or on a treadmill can strengthen your leg, hip and back muscles and help to protect you against osteoarthritis. Strap the weight bands to your ankles, placing one weight in each. Walk a few steps to determine your response. If, later, you feel only slight discomfort, repeat the exercise every day until the discomfort abates. Next, increase the time spent wearing the weight bands, then slowly add more weights. Note, however, that some people may not be able to tolerate this exercise at all.

Grippers

Squeezing cushioned 'hand-grippers' between your thumbs and fingers can greatly increase the strength and dexterity of your hands. Furthermore, almost all people with fibromyalgia will be able to perform this exercise, slowly and steadily increasing the number of repetitions. Hand-grippers can be purchased at most sports shops.

Aerobic exercise

Because the muscles in a person with fibromyalgia are unable to adequately utilize oxygen, aerobic exercise is beneficial. It has actually been proven to significantly reduce the pain and fatigue of the condition. The improvements may be due to the fact that aerobic exercise releases 'feel-good' endorphins – the 'natural' painkillers. In addition, muscle temperature rises, helping muscles to relax, so they receive more oxygen and waste products are removed more efficiently. The cardiovascular system also benefits from aerobic exercise, helping to protect against heart disease, improving circulation and meaning you are less out of breath. Regular aerobic activity also carries the added bonuses of increasing your stamina levels and helping you to lose weight.

The strengthening exercises described above should be performed for at least two weeks before embarking on aerobic activity. The increased muscle capacity that results from them allows greater benefit to be gained from aerobic activity.

Ideally, you should then aim to develop a programme involving a small amount of aerobic activity, preferably of the low-intensity type. Jogging on a hard floor or road, using a rowing machine or any multigym equipment is not recommended in fibromyalgia.

Note: Check with your doctor before going ahead with *any* aerobic activity.

Types of low-impact aerobic activities

The following aerobic activities are listed in order of difficulty. If you feel able to perform more than one, be sure to work through them in the order given.

Walking

Always ensure you choose an aerobic exercise you enjoy and one that is within your physical – and practical – scope. Walking is good. It is a weight-bearing activity that increases mobility, strength, stamina and helps protect against osteoporosis. If your symptoms are severe, you may just want to walk to the nearest lamp post and back on your first day. On the second and third days, you should try to repeat that. On the fourth day, you could try walking to the second lamp post, on the fifth and sixth days to repeat that, on the seventh to the third lamp post, on the ninth and tenth to repeat that and so on. For most people, walking is the easiest and most convenient aerobic activity. You may surprise yourself at how far you actually can walk after increasing the distance over several weeks.

However, you must be wary of walking outdoors in cold, damp conditions. An electrically operated treadmill can, if you can afford the initial outlay, be an excellent investment. It will give you the freedom to walk for as long as you want during winter as well as summer, whatever the weather. Also, as a treadmill offers continuous level walking, people with lower back, hip and leg pain may walk for far greater distances this way than they could hope to over the variable terrain found outdoors. Although some people consider treadmill walking too monotonous and artificial, this can, to some extent, be overcome by positioning it near a shelf so you can read a book or magazine at the same time. Wearing an MP3 player or CD player so you can listen to your favourite music, or listening to the radio or to an audio book passes the time quickly, too. However, this said, treadmills should never wholly replace outdoor walking. Fresh air and sunlight are also important factors in lessening the effects of fibromyalgia.

Stepping

Although greatly beneficial, not everyone with fibromyalgia will be able to perform step exercises. If you think you may be able to manage, you should start with a small step, such as a wide, hefty book or maybe a catalogue or telephone directory. Make sure it is placed securely against a bottom stair to keep it steady and so you have room to move. (After two or three weeks, you may be able to use the bottom stair itself.) Place first your left foot, then your right foot on the book or step. Now step backwards with first your left foot, then your right. Repeat between two and ten times, then alternate your feet, placing first your right foot, then your left. You may eventually be able to perform the exercise for five or ten minutes.

Trampoline jogging

Jogging on a small, circular trampoline can, if care is taken, be good aerobic exercise. Become accustomed to the feel of it by, at first, simply lifting your heels – not your feet – as if you are walking. If you can manage to get into a rhythm, the trampoline will do much of the work for you. Continue for two or three minutes.

Walking on the spot should be your next aim and then gentle jogging a while after that, if you can. Don't get carried away, though! Sharp jolts and jerks may do more harm than good. Small, inexpensive trampolines are available from most sports shops.

Aqua-aerobics

Although swimming can be counter-productive in fibromyalgia, aqua-aerobics, sometimes called 'aqua-cizes', can be a pleasing and beneficial alternative. Because the water supports your body as you exercise – when you are submerged to the neck, you bear only about a tenth of your body weight – it removes the shock factor, conditioning your muscles with the minimum of discomfort. The pressure of the water also causes the chest to expand, encouraging deeper breathing and increased oxygen intake.

Rather than exercising alone in the baths, most people prefer to join an aqua-aerobics class. As well as providing encouragement and ensuring that you exercise properly for maximum benefit, this can bring you into contact with people who have similar health problems, such as arthritis, so you can empathize with, and support, each other. Most public swimming baths run aqua-aerobics sessions, some of which are graded according to ability. You should inform the instructor of your limitations and avoid the more taxing exercises. I would advise that you phone, first of all, to check the water temperature as exercising in water below 29°C (84°F) will cause your muscles to tighten – it may even induce a flare-up.

Aqua-aerobics, as with all types of exercise, is only truly beneficial when performed regularly. If you live a long way from the swimming baths, you will probably find yourself attending less and less as time goes by, then feel angry with yourself for eventually giving up. To minimize feelings of failure, be wary of undertaking activities that it will be hard for you to keep doing regularly.

Cycling

Whether using an exercise bike or an actual bicycle, this activity provides an efficient cardiovascular workout. However, caution must rule. People who suffer from lower back and buttock pain may, despite using a seat cushion, find that cycling aggravates the problem. Often the handlebars are too far forwards, which can heighten neck, shoulder and upper back pain. Also, due to the continuous motion, your legs have no opportunity to rest, as they would between spells of most other types of exercise. Cycling can, therefore, create much pain for later.

It is best to start by pedalling slowly, gradually building momentum and, at first, limit your sessions to two or three minutes. After a month or so, people with milder symptoms may be able to cycle for 20 to 30 minutes. If you use an exercise bike, always set it at a low resistance level.

Cooling-down exercises

Cooling down your muscles after exercise is just as important as warming them up beforehand. The longer stretches described below should only be done when your muscles are sufficiently warm, after exercise. Again, you should choose the exercises with which you know you can cope. If all the following are beyond your scope, repeat your choice of warm-up exercises instead. The cool-down phase should last up to five minutes.

Calves

Keeping your right leg and back straight, place your palms against a wall, then bend your left knee (so that it extends further than your left ankle). Press the heel of your right foot into the floor until you feel a gentle stretch. (Move your right foot further back if you don't feel a stretch.) Now exercise the other calf in the same way.

Upper back

Sitting on the floor, your knees bent, hold on to your ankles and slowly round out your back. Pull in your tummy and lower your head until you feel a gentle stretch in the middle and upper parts of your back.

Chest

Sitting on the floor, place your hands on your lower back, then move your shoulders back until you feel a gentle stretch in your chest (see Figure 17).

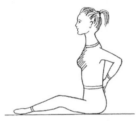

Figure 17 Cooling-down stretch for the chest

Backs of the thighs

Lie on your back, using a small rolled cloth or towel to support your neck, and lift both knees, keeping your feet flat on the floor. Now raise your left leg. Placing one hand behind and above your knee and the other behind and below it, slowly ease the leg towards your shoulders until you feel a gentle stretch along the

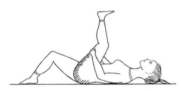

Figure 18 Cooling-down stretch for the backs of the thighs

back of your left thigh. Next, do the same with the right leg (see Figure 18).

Fronts of the thighs

Lying on your stomach, bend your left leg and hold your ankle with your nearest hand.

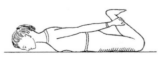

Figure 19 Cooling-down stretch for the fronts of the thighs

Now, keeping your back straight, push your pelvis into the floor until you feel a gentle stretch along the front of your left thigh. Now do the same with the right leg (see Figure 19).

Abdominal muscles

Lying on your stomach, place your hands and forearms on the floor and slowly raise your upper body until you feel a gentle stretch in your abdominal muscles (see Figure 20).

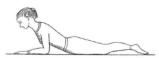

Figure 20 Cooling-down stretch for the abdominal muscles

Other exercises

The exercises 'Back of the upper arms' (Figure 11, page 77) and 'Thighs', (Figures 7, 8 and 9, pages 75–6) should also be included in your cooling-down routine.

Getting started on your routine

First of all, it is advisable to exercise before your pain levels start to rise. It is important, too, that you set aside sufficient time to perform your routine – don't be tempted to rush.

- Relax your muscles by taking a warm shower shortly after waking.
- Eat a light breakfast to boost your energy levels – you should not exercise after a heavy meal.
- Dress in loose, comfortable clothing and good, supportive trainers.
- Ensure that you exercise in a warm place, out of draughts.
- Start slowly and carefully. Be sure to only perform two or three repetitions of your chosen exercises. People with milder symptoms will be able to build up to ten repetitions sooner than people with severe symptoms.
- Movements should be kept within your range. If you know that raising your arms past a certain level gives rise to pain in your shoulder, make sure you don't initially pass that level. You should actually be able to extend your range with time.
- As you exercise, keep checking your posture. When you allow

your head and shoulders to droop, your back to slouch, you put added strain on your muscles. They then burn more energy, causing additional pain and fatigue.

- Take care that you don't involuntarily hold your breath when exercising. Breathe deeply and evenly, breathing out on the effort.
- Try to visualize the muscle group being exercised. This should prevent other muscle groups accidentally being worked.
- Ensure you pause between repetitions. As there is a slight delay between muscle contraction and relaxation, contracting a muscle without pausing means you do so when the muscle has already contracted. This causes a build-up of lactic acid in the area concerned, which, in turn, causes more pain.
- After exercising, it is important to allow time for recovery before attempting further activity. Don't berate yourself if your pain levels are surprisingly high afterwards. Get some extra rest, then begin a toned-down version of your routine as soon as you are able.
- When you finish you should feel as if you could have done more. This should ensure you don't set yourself up for more pain for later.
- Don't try to make up for the days when you weren't able to do much. Set your limit at the start of each session and stick to it.

6

Complementary therapies

I was taking the appropriate medications, my eating habits had improved and I was starting to exercise ... I certainly felt better physically, but I still needed extra help ...

Complementary medicine has been described as all the therapies not taught in medical school. These include acupuncture, aromatherapy, chiropractic, homeopathy, osteopathy and reflexology, among others. You may know these techniques as 'alternative therapies', but this term can be misleading. The word 'alternative' suggests that it can be used to replace conventional medicine. Unfortunately, for chronic pain conditions, this is rarely the case.

Complementary therapies are suitable for people who have chronic pain for the following reasons:

- they are non-invasive;
- they are largely free from side effects;
- they can be used in addition to long-term medication;
- most of them are enjoyable – the 'patient' can often relax completely, especially during the touch and massage techniques.

In a survey I carried out a few years ago on the members of the support group in my area, the most popular complementary therapy was aromatherapy. This was closely followed by reflexology, acupuncture and chiropractic. It seemed that no one had tried homeopathy, acupressure, the Bowen technique, Bach flower remedies or bioelectromagnetic therapy. However, following an introductory speech by a registered homeopathic practitioner and after the questionnaires were completed and returned, several members, including myself, are now finding homeopathic remedies very helpful. I believe that most of the other therapies were not tried simply because they were not readily available.

People who use complementary therapies do report substantial benefits, although some of this may be the result of knowing that they are doing something positive to help themselves. Different techniques seem to suit different people, so try some and see what works best for you.

Acupressure

Acupressure is an ancient form of oriental healing, combining acupuncture and massage. Practitioners of this technique use the thumbs, fingertips or palms of the hands to firmly massage pressure points, located at specific sites throughout the body. These points are the same as those used in acupuncture (see below for more details). Neither oils nor equipment are used in this type of therapy.

Acupressure is believed to enhance the body's own healing mechanisms. Pain relief is sometimes rapid. However, improvements can take longer in chronic pain conditions. At some hospitals in the UK, acupressure is available as part of the physiotherapy treatment options.

Acupuncture

Also an ancient form of oriental healing, acupuncture involves puncturing the skin with fine needles at specific points of the body. These points are located along energy channels (meridians) that are believed to correspond with certain internal organs. This energy is known as *chi*. Needles are inserted to increase, decrease or unblock the flow of *chi* energy so that the balance of yin and yang is restored. Yin, the female force, is calm and passive; it also represents dark, cold, swelling and moisture. On the other hand, yang, the male force, is stimulating and aggressive, representing heat, light, contraction and dryness. It is thought that an imbalance of these forces is the cause of illness and disease. For example, a person who feels the cold and suffers from fluid retention and fatigue would be considered to have an excess of yin. A person suffering from headaches, however, will be deemed to have an excess of yang.

Emotional, physical or environmental factors are believed to disturb the *chi* energy balance, and can also be treated. For example, acupuncture is used to alleviate stress, digestive disorders, insomnia, asthma and allergy. It is also documented as being successful in relieving pain.

A qualified acupuncturist will use a set method to determine which acupuncture points to use – it is thought there are as many as 2,000 acupuncture points on the body. At a consultation, questions will be asked about lifestyle, sleeping patterns, fears, phobias and reactions to stress. The pulses will be felt, then the acupuncture itself carried out. The first consultation will normally last an hour, and patients should feel improvements after four to six sessions.

Acupuncture is now losing its unorthodox reputation, and is generally accepted in the Western world. In recent years, it has gained so much respect in the medical field that many GPs have learned how to perform the therapy (see the Useful addresses section at the back of the book for contact details for the British Acupuncture Council, which can give you more information).

Aromatherapy

Aromatherapy uses our sense of smell in the treatment of certain health disorders. Concentrated aromatic, or essential, oils are extracted from plants and may be inhaled, mixed with a carrier oil and rubbed directly into the skin, or used in bathing. Each scent relates to its plant of origin, so lavender oil has the same scent as the lavender plant and geranium smells like the geranium plant.

Plant essences have been used for healing throughout the ages, smaller amounts being used for aromatherapy purposes than for herbal medicines. The highly concentrated aromatherapy oils are obtained either by steaming a particular plant extract until the oil glands burst or by soaking the plant extract in hot oil so that the cells collapse and release their essence.

Techniques used in aromatherapy
Inhalation

Effecting the quickest result, inhalation of essential oils has a direct influence on the olfactory (nasal) organs and these are immediately received by the brain. Steam inhalation is the most popular technique. This can be achieved either by mixing a few drops of oil with a bowlful of boiling water or by using an oil burner whereby a candle heats a small container full of water to which a few drops of oil have been added.

Massage

Essential oils intended for massage are diluted before use. They should never be applied directly to the skin in an undilute (pure) form. When using undiluted essential oils, mix three or four drops with a neutral carrier oil, such as olive or safflower oil. The oils penetrate the skin and are absorbed by the body, exerting a positive influence on a particular organ or set of tissues.

Bathing

Tension and anxiety can be reduced by using certain aromatherapy oils in the bath. A few drops of one or more pure essential oils should be added directly to running tap water. It mixes more efficiently this way than if it is added after you have turned off the taps. No more than 20 drops of oil in total should be added to bathwater.

Oils for relaxation

Lavender is the most popular oil for relaxation purposes. It is known to be a wonderful restorative and excellent for relieving tension headaches as well as stress. However, there are several others that when used alone or blended can provide a relaxing atmosphere – Roman chamomile and ylang ylang, for example. Ylang ylang has relaxing properties, a calming effect on the heart rate and can relieve palpitations and raised blood pressure. Chamomile can be very soothing, too, and aids both sleep and digestion.

Drop your relaxation oils into the vessel part of an oil burner and top up with water. Light a tea light candle (placed beneath the burner) and try to relax while the essential oils scent the whole room and you inhale their fragrance. Such oils are safe around babies and children, as rather than being overpowering, the aroma is soft and soothing.

Recipe 1

- 5 drops of lavender
- 2 drops of Roman chamomile
- 1 drop of ylang ylang.

Blend well and diffuse in a burner.

Recipe 2

- 8 drops of mandarin
- 3 drops of neroli
- 3 drops of ylang ylang.

Blend well and diffuse in a burner.

Recipe 3

- 10 drops of bergamot
- 2 drops of rose otto
- 3 drops of Roman chamomile.

Blend well and diffuse in a burner.

The oils from either recipe 2 or 3 can be added to two ounces of distilled water, shaken well and used in a spray bottle for a non-toxic room freshener with relaxing properties.

Recipe 4

For relaxation, this is a great blend for use in the bath.

- 3 drops of lavender
- 2 drops of marjoram
- 2 drops of basil
- 1 drop of vetiver
- 1 drop fennel.

Stimulating oils

The aromatherapy oils capable of stimulating mind and body, boosting the immune system and reducing fatigue include orange, rose, lavender and neroli. These oils can be mixed together in different combinations and added to a carrier oil, such as tea tree oil, to make massage oils.

Seeing an aromatherapist

As aromatherapy is an holistic therapy (where the practitioner looks at you and your ills as part of the whole), the aromatherapist is likely to ask questions about lifestyle, family circumstances and so on. Depending on your answers, a suitable essential oil or oils will be chosen and a gentle massage given. As well as being beneficial healthwise, aromatherapy massages are very relaxing.

If you are unable to consult with a qualified aromatherapist, your local healthfood shop may provide you with details of which essential oils are appropriate for your needs. Alternatively, you could borrow a good aromatherapy book from the library (details are given under Further reading at the back of this book).

Bach flower remedies

In the 1930s, the philosophy of a Harley Street doctor, Edward Bach (pronounced 'batch'), was 'a healthy mind ensures a healthy body'. He was a man far ahead of his time, for mind and body are only now being more widely seen as closely linked.

Dr Bach devised a method of treating the negative emotional state behind any disorder. First he sectioned emotional states into seven major groups – such as fear, loneliness, uncertainty – then he categorized 38 negative states of mind under each group. Using his knowledge of homeopathy, he went on to formulate a plant- or flower-based remedy to treat each of these emotional states, as follows:

1 *Fear*
- For terror, he formulated Rock Rose remedy.
- For fear of known things, he formulated Mimulus.
- For fear of mental collapse, he formulated Cherry Plum.
- For fears and worries of unknown origin, he formulated Aspen.
- For fear or overconcern for others, he formulated Red Chestnut.

2 *Loneliness*
- For impatience, he formulated Impatiens.
- For self-centredness/self-concern, he formulated Heather.
- For pride and aloofness, he formulated Water Violet.

3 *Insufficient interest in present circumstances*
- For apathy, he formulated Wild Rose.
- For lack of energy, he formulated Olive.
- For unwanted thoughts/mental arguments he formulated White Chestnut.
- For lack of interest in the present, he formulated Clematis.
- For deep gloom with no known origin, he formulated Mustard.
- For failure to learn from mistakes, he formulated Chestnut Bud.

4 *Despondency or despair*
- For extreme mental anguish, he formulated Sweet Chestnut.
- For self-hatred/sense of uncleanliness, he formulated Crab Apple.
- For overresponsibility, he formulated Elm.
- For lack of confidence, he formulated Larch.
- For self-reproach/guilt, he formulated Pine.
- For after-effects of shock, he formulated Star of Bethlehem.
- For resentment, he formulated Willow.
- For exhausted but struggling on, he formulated Oak.

5 *Uncertainty*
- For hopelessness and despair, he formulated Gorse.
- For despondency, he formulated Gentian.
- For indecision, he formulated Scleranthus.
- For uncertainty as to the correct path in life, he formulated Wild Oat.
- For the seeker of advice and confirmation from others, he formulated Cerato.
- For 'Monday morning' feeling, he formulated Hornbeam.

6 *Oversensitivity to influences and ideas*
- For weak will and subserviency, he formulated Centaury.
- For mental torment behind a brave face, he formulated Agrimony.
- For hatred, envy/jealousy, he formulated Holly.
- For protection from change and outside influences, he formulated Walnut.

7 *Overcareful of the welfare of others*
- For intolerance, he formulated Beech.
- For overenthusiasm, he formulated Vervain.
- For self-repression/self-denial, he formulated Rock Water.
- For the selfishly possessive, he formulated Chicory.

In addition, the Rescue Remedy is appropriate to many everyday situations in which emotional upheaval occurs. It is made from a combination of five Bach flower remedies – Rock Rose, Clematis, Cherry Plum, Impatiens and Star of Bethlehem.

Bioelectromagnetics

Bioelectromagnetics is the study of how living organisms – all of which produce electrical currents – interact with magnetic fields. The electrical currents within our bodies are capable of creating magnetic fields that extend outside our bodies, and these fields can be influenced by external magnetic forces. In fact, specific external magnetism can actually produce physical and behavioural changes. Just as drugs induce a response in their target tissues, so low magnetic fields can produce a chosen biological response, but without the side effects associated with drugs. However, external magnetism should not be used by anyone who has a heart pacemaker.

External magnetism can not only correct abnormalities in the energy fields of patients with disease, effectively working as a healer, it is also capable of stabilizing a chronic condition, although not in every case. As a pain reliever, external magnetism has long been used in the Far East and is becoming ever more widely used and much experimentation is currently taking place. Furthermore, electromagnetic machinery is becoming a regular part of NHS treatment. The machinery creates a pulsed magnetic field that is used to aid the recovery of bone fractures, tendon and ligament tears, muscle injuries and so on. A small, light, comparatively inexpensive version of the above can be purchased for easy-to-wear home use.

When placed directly over the site of aches, pains or injuries, external magnetism is called magnotherapy. The following are examples of magnotherapy products now on the market:

- *Seating* Chairs containing magnets at specific sites are now available. They can help to relax tension and reduce/prevent stiffness arising from prolonged sitting.
- *Massage tools* Claimed to be the fastest-working massage implement, a magnetic massager delivers stimulating vibration that can boost circulation and relax the muscles. The massager can easily be used on painful areas. The magnetic head is battery powered.
- *Mattress pads* Available for one person in a double bed, a magnetic mattress is durable and light enough to take on holiday. Thicker, super-magnetized mattress pads are also available.
- *Pillow pads* Usable as a pillow in bed, as well as for sitting, these pads are light and portable.

Also available are magnetized body, arm/leg, neck, elbow, wrist/ carpal, thumb, back, knee and ankle wraps.

External magnetism in the form of a specially designed wrist appliance, worn like a wrist watch, is also believed to be effective in treating aches, pains and injuries in any region of the body. As with the other types of external magnetism, this appliance is said to improve the ability of the blood to carry oxygen and nutrients around the body. It is also believed to speed the removal of toxins and other waste products.

The Bowen technique

This dynamic system of muscle and connective tissue therapy is revolutionizing pain management (and other healthcare practices) worldwide. Australian Tom Bowen, who pioneered the technique in the 1950s, had successfully treated approximately 13,000 patients annually – with 80 to 90 per cent of them responding favourably after only one or two treatments – before the technique was documented and introduced into other countries. Now widely recognized as a safe and effective therapy, the practitioner performs a sequence of small, precise movements at specific points on the body. This provokes a stimulus that releases the tissues in the problem area(s), which, in turn, triggers the body's own healing mechanisms.

The therapy can be performed through light clothing, while the patient is in a reclined position. A session will normally take 30 to 45 minutes, inclusive of short breaks to allow the body time to adjust to each part of the treatment. The patient will then be asked to drink a litre ($1^3/_4$ pints) of water within the following few hours to aid the removal of toxins from the lymphatic system.

Patients normally find the treatment relaxing and many report almost immediate improvements. Others may feel improvements over the following two or three weeks, as the first treatment takes full effect. Long-standing pain may be eliminated in some conditions after three to six weeks of treatment. In fibromyalgia, the pain can be notably reduced for substantial periods – people with mild symptoms even reporting a total elimination of pain.

The Bowen technique is rapidly gaining in popularity and treatment clinics are being set up throughout the UK (see the Useful addresses section at the back of the book for further details.)

Chiropractic

Chiropractic is a non-invasive therapy used to alleviate pain by muscle manipulation and spinal adjustment. Muscles are held together and connected to the joints by myofascia – a tube-like lining encasing the muscles and attaching them to the bones. The elevated muscle tension prevalent in fibromyalgia may, at times of physical or emotional stress, cause the myofascia to bunch up, impeding the flow of oxygen to the muscle cells. The muscles shorten, straining the myofascia and tendinous attachments, limiting their movement and making them susceptible to tearing (see Chapter 1 for more details).

In short, then, microscopic tears in the muscle fibres are thought to intensify pain and muscle fatigue. This may, in part, also be due to the fact that adjoining muscles are unable to slide over them as easily as they should. Painful trigger points may develop where muscle and bone connect. This circumstance may even pull joints out of position, so much so that they become fixated, which means that the joint will not return to its natural position by itself and is therefore more painful. Chiropractors specializing in soft tissue manipulation (or myofascial pain syndrome techniques) may be helpful in reducing trigger-point pain, tender-point pain and correcting bone misalignments and fixations.

At the initial consultation, a chiropractor will need to thoroughly evaluate your condition. This is normally done with the help of X-rays. Many chiropractors also use the following to treat patients.

- *Ultrasound machines* An ultrasound machine performs a micro-massage of the muscle by producing sound waves that penetrate the tissues. The round applicator is simply moved over the surface of a painful area to help reduce muscle tension and pain. Physiotherapists also use ultrasound.
- *Microcurrent stimulation* This may be used to duplicate the body's own healing frequencies. The stimulator produces a low-voltage microelectrical current that feels like non-painful tingling. This technique should help relax muscles, restore normal circulation to the region and reduce pain. It is considered excellent for reducing jaw pain.
- *Spinal adjustment by hand* is another chiropractic technique, but one with which people with fibromyalgia may not be able to

cope. A spring-loaded activator – a 15.5-cm (6-in) long spring-loaded device – may be used instead. The chiropractor will set a tension level in order to deliver a specific force. The tension should be low for people with fibromyalgia.

- *Massage* may also be performed by a chiropractor. However, the chiropractor should take care to be gentle and not aggravate muscles that are already sore.

Finding the right chiropractor

A chiropractor needs to know about fibromyalgia if he or she is to help rather than hurt you. Thus, before booking any sessions, it is important that you ask the following basic questions:

- 'Do you understand what fibromyalgia is?' If the answer is 'yes', ask the remaining questions.
- 'Are you aware that spinal adjustment can hurt people with fibromyalgia?' If the answer is 'yes', ask how this problem can be avoided.
- 'Do you use X-rays in your initial assessment?'
- 'What methods do you use – ultrasound, microcurrent stimulation and others?'
- 'Do you offer help in devising an exercise programme?'

It is imperative that the chiropractor you choose answers each of the above questions to your satisfaction. At your first consultation, ensure the chiropractor understands your full medical history – many people with fibromyalgia have a lengthy medical background. Remind your chiropractor to be gentle as often as required and ensure you speak up if a particular treatment hurts. (See the Useful addresses section at the back of the book for contact details for the British Chiropractic Association.)

Herbal remedies

When modern medicines (prescription drugs) were developed in the twentieth century, people decided they were more effective than herbs and that the latter were simply 'old wives' tales' that really didn't work. However, traditional Chinese herbal remedies have been used, to great effect, since antiquity and in fact 30 per cent of prescription drugs are made from plant-derived substances. Herbs are the natural choice, though, with far less risk of side effects than prescription drugs. They should still be used with caution as they can interact with prescription drugs. If you would like to try using herbal remedies, inform your doctor before starting treatment. Remember that as herbs work at a slower pace than prescription drugs, you must have patience. Indeed, it can take up to four months for fibromyalgia treatments to start showing benefits. You should also be aware that herbal remedies will not help if your body is deficient in certain nutrients. You need to try your best, therefore, to eat a healthy balanced diet with plenty of fruit and vegetables, grains, pulses, nuts and so on (see the Further reading section at the back of this book for details of fibromyalgia diet books).

If you prefer to visit a herbalist, your pulse rate and the colour of your tongue will first be checked for clues as to which bodily organs are depleted of energy. You will then be given a prescription for very precise doses according to your needs. Tablets made from compressed herbal extracts are sometimes offered, but you may instead be given a bag of carefully weighed and ground dried roots, flowers, bark and so on. In the latter case, an 'infusion' should be made by pouring boiled water directly on to the herbal mixture. It should be covered and left to stand for 10 to 30 minutes, maybe stirring occasionally. The resulting liquid should then be strained and drunk.

The following herbs are known to be useful in treating some of the symptoms of fibromyalgia.

Ginkgo biloba

Many studies have been carried out on *Ginkgo biloba* and its effectiveness is now well documented. When used in the treatment of fibromyalgia, this herb can help maintain and support the body's circulation, particularly to the extremities (the hands and feet) and, most importantly, the brain. The advantages include better cerebral blood flow, improved tissue oxygenation, more efficient energy production and improved cognitive function in terms of concentration and short-term memory.

In a 1992 trial, volunteers were given doses of 40 mg of *Ginkgo biloba* three times a day. After one month, their short-term memories had improved noticeably. In another trial, 600-mg doses were given daily. The volunteers experienced even sharper reactions and better memories, without side effects, indicating improved brain functioning, all of which was judged to be due to improved circulation. *Ginkgo biloba* is, therefore, considered useful in the treatment of fibromyalgia.

St John's wort

St John's wort is probably the most successful natural antidepressant. Studies have shown that it works by increasing the action of the chemical serotonin (as noted earlier, people with fibromyalgia normally have low levels of available serotonin) and by inhibiting depression-promoting enzymes. Similar effects are created by the Prozac and Nardil families of orthodox antidepressants, but both have a high risk of side effects. St John's wort, however, has the happy advantage of being virtually free of side effects. In some cases it can produce a stomach upset, but this should stop within a few days.

St John's wort is believed to encourage sleep and benefit the immune system. In Germany, this herb outsells Prozac by three to one and is said to be just as effective. St John's wort also has anti-inflammatory properties. It helps fight viral infections, too. For it to have its full effect typically takes two weeks.

Note: Because your skin may be more sensitive to the sun's rays when you are taking this herb, don't forget to use a good sunblock.

Other useful remedies

Chamomile – this herb can help to induce sleep and reduce anxiety.
Cayenne – tension headaches and migraines can be eased with this herb. When made into a salve or ointment, it can relieve muscle pain, too.
Ginseng – this herb boosts energy and relieves stress. If buying in supplement form, look for a good brand as some ginseng extract is not absorbed by the body very well.
Lavender – depression, insomnia, anxiety and headaches can be relieved with this herb.
Milk thistle – this herb supports the liver and improves the immune system and endocrine system (hormones).
Passion flower – this herb helps to combat insomnia, anxiety and stress.

Turmeric – pain and inflammation can be reduced with this herb.
Willow bark – this herb has anti-inflammatory properties and is useful as a painkiller.

Homeopathy

The homeopathic approach to medicine is holistic – that is, your overall health, your physical, emotional and psychological well-being, is assessed before treatment commences. The homeopathic belief is that the whole make-up of a person determines the disorders to which that person is prone, and the symptoms likely to occur. After a thorough consultation, the homeopath will offer a remedy that is compatible with your symptoms as well as your temperament and characteristics. Consequently, two people with the same disorder may be offered entirely different remedies.

Homeopathic remedies are derived from plant, mineral and animal substances, which are soaked in alcohol to extract what are known as the 'live' ingredients. This initial solution is then diluted many times, being vigorously shaken to add energy at each dilution. Impurities are removed and the remaining solution made up into tablets, ointments, powders or suppositories. Low-dilution remedies are used for severe symptoms, while high-dilution remedies are used for milder symptoms.

The homeopathic concept has, since antiquity, been that 'like cures like'. The full healing abilities of this type of remedy were first recognized in the early nineteenth century when a German doctor, Samuel Hahnemann, noticed that the herbal cure for malaria – which was based on an extract of cinchona bark (quinine) – actually produced symptoms of malaria. Further tests convinced him that the production of mild symptoms caused the body to fight the disease. He went on to successfully treat malaria patients with dilute doses of cinchona bark.

Each homeopathic remedy has first been 'proved' by being taken by healthy people – usually volunteer homeopaths – and the symptoms noted. The remedy is then known to be capable of curing the same symptoms in an ill person. The whole idea of 'proving' and using homeopathic remedies can be difficult to understand, especially as it is exactly the opposite of how conventional medicines operate. For example, in homeopathy, a patient who has a cold with a runny nose would be treated with a remedy that would produce a runny nose in a healthy patient. Conventional medicine, on the other hand, would provide something that dries up the nose in a healthy or well person.

Nowadays, a homeopathic remedy can be formulated to aid virtually every disorder. Although remedies are safe and non-addictive, occasionally the patient's symptoms may briefly worsen. This is known as a 'healing crisis' and is usually short-lived. It is actually a good indication that the remedy is working well.

You should visit a homeopath if you have a medical problem that is not getting better or if you are constantly swapping one set of symptoms for another. It is a common misconception that you can just pop along to your local chemist, look up your particular complaint on the homeopathic remedy chart and begin taking the remedy. If only it were that simple. Homeopathic training takes several years and a lot of knowledge and experience is required before practitioners can decide the correct remedies for complaints other than the very superficial. Also, as mentioned earlier, what works for one person will not always work for another, so a proper consultation is essential.

Selecting an appropriate remedy is only part of the procedure, however. The homeopath will also evaluate patient reaction to ascertain what, if any, further treatment is necessary. People who use prescribed homeopathic remedies generally notice a rapid improvement in their condition.

Hydrotherapy

I thought it appropriate here to mention a self-help therapy that can be done at home. As most of us are already aware, a long soak in a hot bath is profoundly relaxing. It also has a wonderfully calming effect on the central nervous system.

Even more soothing, surprisingly, is a long soak in a bath as close as possible to body temperature (36.1°C, 96.9°F). For best results, the bathwater should cover your shoulders and the longer you are immersed, the better you will feel. For comfort, place a folded towel behind your head. The water should provide adequate support, though, as a body in water weighs only a quarter of its normal weight. Keep the temperature of the water as constant as possible by regularly topping-up from the hot tap.

Hypnotherapy

Hypnotherapy may be described as psychotherapy using hypnosis. There is, however, still no acceptable definition of the actual state of hypnosis. It is commonly described as an altered state of consciousness, lying somewhere between being awake and asleep. People under hypnosis are aware of their surroundings, yet their minds are, to a large extent, under the control of the hypnotist. People under hypnosis also seem to pass control of their actions, as well as a portion of their thoughts, to the hypnotist. We have all seen people under hypnosis on TV, acting out a role. At the time they are absorbed in what they have been 'told' to do – often instigated by a specific 'trigger' word – but immediately afterwards they wonder what on earth they were up to. Their behaviour had been dictated, to a certain degree, by the hypnotist. There is no need to worry as hypnotherapy is about the hypnotist using this power for therapeutic purposes rather than entertainment!

Hypnotherapy is performed by putting the patient into a 'trance'. By the early nineteenth century, some physicians were using hypnotism – then called 'mesmerism' – to perform pain-free operations. The majority of the medical profession were highly sceptical, however, believing the patients to have been either schooled or paid to show no pain. Not until the last two decades did hypnotism become an accepted form of therapy.

Nowadays, a hypnotherapist takes a full psychological and physiological history of each patient, then slowly talks him or her into a trance state. The therapist can use either direct suggestion – by indicating that the patient's pain, for example, will notably lessen – or begin to explore the root cause of any tension, anxiety or depression. Of course, where fibromyalgia is concerned, physical pain is present as well as certain psychological problems. Hypnotherapy can, therefore, be very helpful.

Hypnotherapists have found that when, in chronic pain conditions, the level of tension is lowered, many of the physical symptoms are also greatly reduced. Some experts in the field believe that the main purpose of hypnotherapy is to aid relaxation, reduce tension and increase the person's confidence and ability to cope with problems.

One common fear is that the therapist may, while the patient is in a trance, implant dangerous suggestions or extract improper personal information. I can only say that a trance is not a wholly stable condition. Patients can come out of it at any time – particularly if they are asked to do or say anything they would not even contemplate when awake. Malpractice would only have to be detected once to ruin the therapist's career. Still, if you are at all worried, go to a recommended hypnotherapist.

Massage

Massage therapy was one of the earliest treatments used by humankind. It enjoyed only average popularity, however, until the nineteenth century, when a Swedish athlete found that a combination of massage and exercise greatly relaxed muscles and joints. This therapy became far more popular when, in 1970, George Dowling's *The Massage Book* (Penguin) was published. It introduced the concept of a holistic approach to the whole technique of massage. Nowadays, your emotional and psychological state, as well as your physical state, is often assessed at the initial consultation.

A good massage helps a person to feel relaxed, both physically and mentally. It is useful in treating depression and anxiety as well as headaches, stiffness, muscle pain and circulatory disorders. It is not, however, appropriate for people suffering inflammation of the veins (phlebitis), varicose veins or thrombosis. Your GP will tell you whether or not you are a suitable candidate, and may even supply details of a qualified therapist.

The massage itself comprises the actions of stroking, drumming, kneading and/or friction (sometimes called 'pressure'). Each of these methods may be used separately or in combination, depending on the patient's symptoms. For people with fibromyalgia, it is advisable, first of all, to enquire whether or not the practitioner is familiar with the condition. Stroking and gentle kneading techniques may be acceptable, but drumming and friction massage might aggravate your symptoms. For some people with the condition, even a light pressure massage can be sufficient to induce severe pain. It is important, therefore, that you speak up if the therapist begins to hurt you.

After a request by the Fibromyalgia Network USA for feedback on the subject of massage therapy, 300 letters were received. An overwhelming majority praised the treatment, many saying that if their budgets allowed, they would have weekly therapy. Because deep massage techniques were often too painful to tolerate, however, most respondents began with some form of 'light touch' therapy. People with severe symptoms started out with a partial body massage (neck, shoulders and back), many leading up to a full-body massage as their toleration increased.

Usually, if you want a massage, you will have to travel to a massage clinic, but some practitioners do make home visits. You may be asked to undress, leaving on only your pants or briefs. If this makes you feel uneasy, you should insist that another person be present. Nowadays, practitioners often combine treatment with aromatherapy, acupuncture or reflexology.

After therapy, many people report an increase in function and a reduction of fatigue. It's important to rest afterwards to ensure that loosened muscles do not immediately re-knot. It is unwise to carry a heavy load of shopping home just because you feel better, for example. Where muscles have successfully been released, you may have soreness for up to two days afterwards. Rest will help ensure that a delayed pain response is minimized.

For sore post-massage muscles, place an ice pack (gel packs that can be both frozen and heated can be purchased at most chemists) on the affected areas. Alternating between cold and heat can be even more beneficial. Taking a warm bath later that evening, maybe with a teaspoonful of Epsom salts, can also help reduce any post-massage soreness.

For those who feel competent and wish to massage someone at home, ensure that the room is warm and peaceful and lay the recipient on a comfortable but firm surface. A pillow placed beneath the upper torso may help to relax the upper back. Massage oil (aromatherapy oils are good) makes the act of massage easier, and hand movements should be smooth, gentle and continuous. Continue the therapy for two or three minutes only, to ensure there are no unwelcome after-effects. If all is well, gradually increase the length of the sessions.

Your local library should carry several books on the subject of massage techniques, many of them including advice on self-massage. Alternatively, you could purchase an electric massager, which you may be able to use yourself. To ease discomfort in more inaccessible areas, ask a friend or partner to help out.

Reflexology

Reflexology, an ancient oriental therapy, has only relatively recently been adopted in the Western world. It works on the principle that the body is divided into different energy zones, represented in different parts of the feet, all of which can be exploited in the prevention and treatment of any disorder.

Reflexologists have identified ten energy channels, which run from the toes and extend to the fingers and the top of the head. Each channel relates to a particular bodily zone, and to the organs in that zone. For example, the big toe relates to the head – the brain, sinus area, neck, pituitary glands, eyes and ears. By applying pressure to the appropriate terminal in the form of a specialized massage, a practitioner can determine which energy pathways are blocked. Minute lumps – like crystalline deposits – detected beneath the skin are then broken down by steady pressure. The theory is that the deposits are absorbed into the body's waste disposal system and eliminated in sweat or urine, hence restoring the correct energy flow.

Experts in this type of manipulative therapy claim that reflexology aids the removal of waste products and blockages within the energy channels, improving circulation and the functioning of the glands. Reflexology is certainly relaxing – indeed, many patients fall asleep during therapy. Because my own feet are so ticklish, I felt I had cause to worry before my first reflexology session. However, I quickly found that the sensations were pleasurable and I was able to relax. I must say, I was surprised to note how accurate the therapist was in detecting my own 'indispositions'.

Many therapists prefer to take down a full case history before commencing treatment. Each session takes up to 45 minutes (the preliminary session will take longer) and you will be treated either sitting in a chair or lying down, depending on both therapist and patient.

Yoga in fibromyalgia

Just five to ten minutes a day of yoga can have surprising benefits for the individual with fibromyalgia, increasing suppleness, a sense of relaxation and general well-being. Yoga is believed to have a calming effect on the body's stress systems and to balance activity in the autonomic nervous system (ANS), which controls our unconscious bodily functions, such as the heart, liver, intestines and other internal organs. A study by Dr Patrick Randolph at Texas Tech University found that gentle yoga stretches and mindfulness meditation improved the ability to cope with chronic pain and, when combined with medication, improved pain symptoms significantly better than drug therapy alone.

One study in 2011 looked at the effects of yoga on levels of cortisol, the hormone produced by the adrenal gland when we are under stress, in women with fibromyalgia. Lead author Kathryn Curtis of York University, Toronto, found that levels of cortisol dropped, as did levels of pain. Participants also reported improvement in other symptoms, as well as psychological benefits such as increased hope, acceptance and sense of empowerment. In particular, the women reported an increased level of mindfulness, or non-judgemental living in the moment, whereby they were better able to detach from agitation, pain and despondency.

Some practitioners, such as Dr Timothy McCall, the author of *Yoga as Medicine* (Bantam Dell, 2007) <www.DrMcCall.com>, also believe that yoga may have a beneficial effect on the brain and unhelpful or unhealthy habits of thought. In line with current thinking about the brain, neuroplasticity (or the belief that the brain is not a fixed structure, but malleable) means that new thoughts and actions can rewire your brain. With time and repeated practice, yoga asanas or postures can introduce healthier thought patterns, strengthening the new neural networks and helping banish old, unhelpful ways of thinking.

Practising yoga

Take it easy – don't rush headlong into it. The general rule is to start very small and build up slowly. Never force your body, and if you experience pain, stop at once. Do not aim for contorted postures or strenuous forms of yoga which may make you feel terrible the next day or even be a risk of injury, especially to the neck and back. Yoga is not an endurance exercise or a challenge to be mastered but a form of gentle stretching which, performed slowly and with all due respect for your tender points, can help relieve the pain of fibromyalgia.

If, like many people with fibromyalgia, you experience morning stiffness, do be careful about when you practise. Allow yourself time to warm up before you try any postures. Some people are not ready before mid-morning or even lunchtime. A warm bath may help, and a warm room in which to practise. Be especially careful of postures involving the back and neck, and be sure to do any recommended warm-up exercises. If you attend a class, tell the instructor you have fibromyalgia.

For those whose symptoms are severe, even the gentler forms of yoga can be too much at the beginning. Try doing postures lying down – or maybe even in a warm bath – or sitting in a chair, until you recover flexibility and strength. Start with exercises for hands and feet – again, some people find it helpful to do these in a bowl of warm water if their extremities are very stiff. I must stress again how important it is to go slowly. Give it time, and don't be daunted by apparent lack of progress. Basic deep breathing, stretching and relaxation exercises can go a long way towards calming a sensitized, stressed nervous system and making you feel comfortable in your body again.

Music therapy

Music is well documented to have a positive effect on chronic pain. In 2013, in the first large-scale review of 400 research papers in the neurochemistry of music, a team led by Professor Daniel J. Levitin of McGill University, Montreal, showed that both playing and listening to music improve mood and have clear benefits for mental and physical health. Professor Levitin and his colleague Dr Mona Lisa Chanda found that the neurochemical effects of music include a reduction in the stress hormone cortisol, as well as in muscle tension and heart rate.

In a 2011 study, a team at the University of Granada, Spain, found that music therapy significantly reduces pain, depression and anxiety, and improves sleep in those with fibromyalgia. Dr María Dolores Onieva-Zafra and colleagues applied a relaxation technique based on guided imagery along with music therapy, and participants were given a CD to listen to at home.

Another study in 2005 by Dr Sandra L. Siedlecki from the Cleveland Clinic Foundation, Ohio, found that listening to music can reduce chronic pain and depression by up to 25 per cent and make people feel more in control and less disabled by their condition. Participants had a range of conditions including osteo-arthritis, disc problems and rheumatoid arthritis. They were either invited to choose their own music, which ranged from pop to slow tunes and nature sounds, or given a relaxing tape featuring piano, jazz, orchestra, harp and synthesizer. Either was effective – whereas the control group showed no improvement in symptoms at all.

Pet therapy

Animal-assisted therapy is increasingly popular as a complementary approach to helping people with a wide range of medical conditions. Obviously, pets are classic stress-relievers, but studies featuring specially trained animals also show they boost the body's production of endorphins and other neurotransmitters, which help fight pain, boost mood and strengthen the immune system.

A study on therapist-trained dogs with fibromyalgia patients at a Pittsburgh pain clinic showed a significant reduction in pain severity after a therapy dog visit, along with improvements in fatigue, stress levels, calmness and cheerfulness. In the study by neurologist Dr Dawn Marcus, late of the University of Pittsburgh, patients were assessed in the waiting room in the 10 to 15 minutes before their doctor's appointment. Pain relief was reported in 34 per cent of the fibromyalgia patients after the dog visit, while, sadly, for those in the waiting room group excluded from the comforts of pet therapy, cheerfulness and fatigue became worse as time increased.

7

Pain and stress management

I'd love to be able to pour out my heart when someone asks how I am! I'd love to be able to say how scared and useless I feel! But I daren't. I don't want to be thought a self-pitying wimp! ... Oh, if only I could find some way of managing all the emotions whirling around in my head, of getting people to believe in me!

Fibromyalgia can affect every area of our lives. In the early stages of the illness, we are often beset by fears for the future, anxieties about our effectiveness as 'functioning' human beings and even doubts about our sanity. Negative feedback from others is also a major source of upset. However, given time, education and self-awareness training, we can gradually adapt to the illness, finding ways to effectively cope with the pain, stress and reactions of others. Just as importantly, we can learn to focus on the present, recapturing feelings of achievement by acquiring new interests, and maybe even a new, more fulfilling career. All these things go a long way towards enhancing quality of life.

A chronic illness

Many people fail to appreciate that any chronic illness – fibromyalgia included – creates problems within the mind as well as the body. Feelings of unreality, vulnerability, guilt, uselessness, fear and of being out of control taint our dealings with others and can be incredibly difficult to shake off.

'I feel so unsure of myself'

The complexity of fibromyalgia can, particularly in the early months/years of the illness, give rise to much self-doubt. When we have pain that, like a ghost, mysteriously transfers from one area to another, when diagnostic tests indicate that everything is fine and when doctors as well as those closest to us stare suspiciously as we describe our unusual symptoms, we may start to wonder if our problems really are of the mind rather than the body!

The fear of mental illness is very real in us all, but to believe it to be a possibility is terrifying. Losing control of our minds means losing connection with ourselves and the world we live in. Threats to our rationality can, ironically, cause emotional problems – stress, anxiety and depression – all of which are far from helpful to our overall state of mind!

Doctors who fail to understand the effects of chronic illness on the individual – especially where there is no validifying diagnosis – invariably amplify these problems. Even after the diagnosis, they can compound the situation by failing to provide information about the disease, neglecting to offer guidance on self-help coping techniques and omitting to outline different treatment options. Unable to cope with the patient's ensuing despair, the doctor is then likely to refer the patient to the psychologist. Sadly, this only serves to endorse the patient's suspicions that he or she has mental problems.

'I feel so vulnerable'

Vulnerability is a natural human condition. We all need people to love us; we all crave the affirmation of others. To a large extent, we are all dependent on others, measuring their responses in order to reassure ourselves that we are worthwhile human beings, that we are indeed loveable. When we are chronically ill, as well as feeling unattractive, we believe we have little to offer the people around us and so fear we are no longer loveable.

Feelings of vulnerability will always be present in chronic illness, but we can defeat the worst of them by looking less to outsiders for affirmation. We all have inner strengths and particular talents, though we may be unware of many of them. Yet, if we waited for others to point them out we would likely be waiting forever!

Your particular forte may be in planning and organizing or problem solving or handling finances – not necessarily out of the family setting. You may be an authority on steam engines, an inspired cook, a good listener, a talented artist, an excellent singer, a diligent student, a competent driver ... so do not underestimate yourself!

'I feel so guilty'

Feelings of guilt are common in chronic illness. It is natural to want to lay the blame for falling ill at someone's door and many of us imagine we ourselves must have done something very wrong to deserve such retribution. Blaming either ourselves or others, though, is pointless. Life is a lottery. Some people are rich, some poor; some clever, some not so clever; some fall ill, some remain healthy. That's just the way it is.

You may, after learning that improvement lies mainly in your hands, feel guilty if you are making no real progress. However, assuming you have tried to help yourself, there is probably a sound reason for your failure. For example, you may have been unable to find information about exactly how to help yourself, be held back by additional health problems or not have allowed sufficient time for any improvements to show.

Pain flare-ups are a perpetual threat in fibromyalgia. Although they can result from 'outside' influences – the weather, a fall, a family crisis – it is likely that a chosen activity caused the exacerbation of pain. So you feel guilty. Viewing a flare-up as a 'painful' learning experience may be some consolation. You attempted to clean the cooker, but afterwards you were rigid with pain. It was a hard lesson but you learned that cleaning the cooker is bad for you!

Guilt also arises when we feel we are a burden on our families. We feel bad about their extra workload and because their free time is now so limited. When people with fibromyalgia need 'full-time' carers, it is important that the carers have time to themselves, that they retain certain interests and have occasional time off. The knowledge that they are enjoying their lives regardless of your ill health and limitations – which, of course, they have a perfect right to do – should help you feel less guilty.

'I feel so afraid'

Of course we are afraid when we have an illness for which there is, as yet, no absolute cure. Our fears tend to centre on the future and what will become of us. We are afraid of being in constant pain, of deteriorating further, of becoming entirely dependent on others, of the long-term effects of medication, that we will lose all our friends ... the list is endless.

Chronic illness exerts profound effects on the individual. It is not always easy to be cheerful and bright when you have a cold, never mind a painful, energy-sapping illness you can see no end to. At least you know that the cold will soon pass, at least you can tell yourself that your spirits will then be restored. Unfortunately, people with fibromyalgia cannot comfort themselves in this way.

However, in most cases of fibromyalgia, the fear of the unknown abates with time. We learn we can take pleasure from family life, enjoy social occasions, take up interests and hobbies and be of use to others. Most importantly, we learn that our condition really can improve – there is no evidence to suggest that fibromyalgia is a degenerative disease. In realizing that the majority of our fears are unfounded, we can get on with our lives more cheerfully.

'I feel so useless'

Fibromyalgia is, without doubt, a limiting condition. Tasks that were once accomplished with ease have, after the onset of the illness, either to be performed with caution or dropped altogether. More often than not, many tasks around the house have to be allocated to other family members or to a paid cleaner. Onlookers may quip, 'Lucky you – having someone else do all the hard work!' They don't realize you would give anything to be able to clean the house thoroughly each and every day.

It is the same with many of the activities you previously enjoyed – and not necessarily ones requiring much effort. For example, some of us are unable to tilt our heads to read or write, and knitting, sewing, sketching, even such a trivial task as filling the kettle, can cause similar problems and may have to be set aside for the present.

Don't give up hope of ever again being able to do the things you enjoyed, though. The heaviest and most 'stretching' of tasks may be permanently out of your scope, but other pleasures (and tasks) can be achieved given time and patience and by the employment of pain- and stress-management strategies (see the end of this chapter). The early months/years of illness are by far the most forbidding, but later you may find you are able to do many of the things you thought you had to set aside forever.

'I feel so out of control'

Having little control over your fibromyalgia is frightening, but, again, this feeling is, as with many other problems, exaggerated during the early months/years. Attempts at regaining a sense of control by, for example, dishing out orders from your sick bed or interfering in other people's lives are not a good idea, however!

In time, we generally evolve our own coping strategies – we may not even be aware of many of them – and learn how to master certain problem situations. We may even end up having more control over our lives than beforehand! For example, we can learn to control the way we talk to and respond to others, train our minds to focus on the present instead of the future, discipline ourselves to take disappointments in our stride and control our viewpoints, developing a more positive, realistic approach to life.

An invisible illness

The thoughtlessness and distrust of others creates difficulties for all people with invisible illness. Even our nearest and dearest can, during a careless moment, say something hurtful. The reason? Simply because they cannot measure our pain, fatigue, anxiety and, for a moment, have failed to bring to mind all we have told them.

When, however, the greater part of their behaviour indicates their concern, we can forgive that momentary lapse. We get upset, though, when others fail to make the same effort, when they show no interest in how we feel or when they interpret our 'behaviour' as weakness. Getting upset serves no useful purpose, however. It only increases the tension in our already painful muscles; it only amplifies stress.

Most people are spurred into activity at the sight of, say, a traffic accident. Instinctively forming a team, the 'onlookers' each play a part in trying to help the injured, making them as comfortable as possible, warning and diverting approaching traffic and alerting the emergency services. Urgency and compassion galvanize them into action. In some instances, onlookers go so far as to put their own lives at risk in their determination to help a person – or even an animal – in trouble. However, those same people are rarely galvanized into action when the crisis is not manifest, when someone suffering from an invisible illness complains of pain or exhaustion.

'Why do people distrust what I say?'

Suspicion arises when, as in fibromyalgia, pain cannot be quantified. Onlookers are unable to see the pain, neither can they see any of the hotchpotch of symptoms of which the person is complaining. In fact, they have never heard of fibromyalgia, so how can it be that bad? Pain that mysteriously travels from one area to another – stomach problems and itching one day, exhaustion and migraine the next – what kind of an illness is that? You have to admit, fibromyalgia is not the easiest of conditions for others to accept.

The people who are trusting and compassionate by nature are usually the first to accept invisible illness in others; they are often the first to offer a friendly ear as well as practical help and advice. Those who spend time with people who have fibromyalgia gradually see for themselves how limited their lives have become, how they have ceased activities they formerly enjoyed. That is down to what is visible.

It is human nature to be suspicious and, sadly, some onlookers are quick to tag people with fibromyalgia as soft, inadequate attention-seekers. Being judged in this way is upsetting, especially when, in most instances, the reverse is actually true. Experts now believe that most people with fibromyalgia play down their symptoms. Among the myriad reasons for this, unfortunate experiences with others leads the field.

Few of you will not have endured boredom, embarrassment or disbelief as you attempted to explain your symptoms to someone enquiring after your health. You may, as a result, have got into the habit of muttering, 'I'm not too bad, thanks' or 'A bit better today …', but, unfortunately, playing down a little-known condition such as fibromyalgia can actually come across as indecision about whether or not you are feeling ill at all! Furthermore, being uncertain of your limitations and giving vague, half-hearted responses only serve to moisten any seeds of doubt already planted in the other person's mind.

It sounds like you can't win, doesn't it? Conveying the nature, severity and complexity of fibromyalgia is, without doubt, incredibly hard work. However, if you are not straightforward, open and brief – listeners get bored when people harp on about their illness – certain people around you may never understand.

'How can I make people understand?'

Sarcastic and derisory remarks from others can chip away at your confidence. They should not, therefore, pass unchallenged. Standing up for yourself is not easy, but doing so can have a releasing effect – the opposite of how you feel when you fake indifference or clam up and walk away. In such instances, you may end up feeling hurt, offended, and very resentful. Your most intense feeling, however, is likely to be that of anger – towards the other person and yourself, for allowing yourself to be hurt.

For example, if your partner were to complain, 'I do all the housework while you do nothing', I suggest you respond, 'I'm trying as hard as I can, but when I have a flare-up, everything I do makes me worse. I know it seems unfair when you're stuck with all the housework ... Maybe it will help you to know that seeing you so busy upsets me, too. I really do appreciate your efforts, though. Perhaps we should learn to put up with a bit of dust and clutter.' If the initial comment was made during a heated exchange, you could answer, 'That's a hurtful thing to say. I may be doing very little, but it's not my fault. I'd like to talk this through when we're calmer.'

When family members are consistently sceptical of your condition – no matter what words or manner you employ – you may be so hurt you consider cutting yourself off from them completely. If their condemnations of you border on the fanatical, then this is perhaps your only choice. Otherwise, you would be best advised to keep steadily hammering away at your case, remembering to bring all unfair comments to their attention.

It may help you to know that when those close remain deaf to your assertions of ill health, it is often because they can't face the fact that their child/partner/parent/sibling/best friend is very ill. The only way they can deal with your illness is to refuse to believe in it. In effect, they cope by not coping. However, that is their problem, not yours. Don't ever give up on them, for almost everything changes with time.

Sadly, people outside your immediate circle of friends/relatives are often capable of being as cutting as the people close to you. Again, they have no right to hurt you, and should not get away with it. Your best weapons here are words that make them think. For example, a person who asks mockingly, 'Are we any better today?' could be answered with, 'Is there something on your mind?

If so, just say it ... If you really are concerned about my health, thank you. The truth is my back is hurting terribly and I don't know how I'll manage to get home.'

People with fibromyalgia frequently face remarks such as, 'I noticed you went shopping last Saturday. I thought you weren't able to walk far!' or 'I saw you in the pub on Saturday night. You must be feeling better!' In such situations, replies could be along the lines of 'Yes, I did manage to get out last weekend. I have good days and bad. But even though I was feeling better, I had to spend two days in bed afterwards.'

'Why have I lost so many friends?'

As you may already have discovered, having fibromyalgia leaves you in little doubt as to who your real friends are. The 'friends' who are offended when you break an appointment, the 'friends' who are unconvinced when you explain that yes you were able to have a night out with them last week, but you feel too ill to go out tonight and worse still the 'friends' who complain that you have again let them down are really not worth your precious energies. Their negative input into your life is detrimental to your confidence as well as to your health.

Guilt is a natural consequence of letting people down. The feeling is amplified when you regularly renege on pre-arranged activities. The ill feeling you know it engenders in others may spur you into attempting activities you know will make you suffer. You may turn up at the next social event despite feeling particularly 'delicate', despite knowing that doing so may provoke a flare-up. Placing yourself at risk in this way is really not worth the fact that you have temporarily assuaged your guilt.

What about the 'friends' who, after you have been unable to socialize as before, have gradually dropped out of your life? Can you honestly say they were true friends? Wouldn't a true friend make allowances for your illness? Wouldn't a true friend try to understand what you are going through?

'Why do people make me feel so upset?'

Even if everyone were charming and accepting around us, fibromyalgia would be a frustrating, upsetting, anger-making business. The reactions of some of the people in our lives only serve to intensify these feelings. We know the condemnation someone who is frequently off sick from work receives. We may even have previously thought badly of someone who regularly complained of ill health. We know that society in general is contemptuous of both mental and physical weakness. When we become ill, all this knowledge seems to form a tight ball in our heads. It only takes one careless comment and we either explode in rage or feel so upset and despairing we want to hide ourselves away.

Without doubt, some people are incredibly insensitive. We may feel we are always on our guard, dreading the remark that will send us into a whirl of anger or spiralling to the depths of despair. Sadly, chronic invisible illness lays us wide open to the misunderstandings of others. As I said earlier, hurtful comments should always be pointed out. If the perpetrator appears contrite, go on to briefly explain just how the illness affects you.

Dealing with negative thinking

Much negative thinking arises from early conditioning. For example, the children of parents who consistently make the same type of comment often grow up with similar basic attitudes. If a woman regularly scoffs at weakness or if her husband or partner repeatedly declares that incompetence is unforgivable, their children have a fair chance of growing up believing this way of thinking is valid and proper.

When people frequently voice negative thoughts, it generally means they are afraid of the very thing about which they are being negative. The mother who decries weakness does it because she secretly fears she is weak. It is the same with the father who denounces incompetence. His attitude stems from deep-seated doubts about his own competence. When their offspring copy these attitudes into adulthood, condemning weakness and incompetence as well as displaying other negative viewpoints, this, too, stems from inherent beliefs that they are lacking in many ways.

Our mindsets – that is, approaching life with an attitude of either trust or distrust, enthusiasm or depression, self-assurance or timidity, anxiety or serenity and so on – usually arise from childhood conditioning. Our automatic thoughts are, therefore, determined by whatever mindsets are built into our character, controlling our behaviour in any given situation. For example, when planning a birthday party, a person with a depressive mindset would dread the 'big day', worrying that few guests would even turn up. A person with an enthusiastic mindset, on the other hand, would eagerly await the party, sure of its success. A person with a trustful mindset would take 'That sweater's a bit small for you' as a caring remark and happily change into something that fitted better. Those with a distrustful mindset, on the other hand, would take it as a criticism of their weight, the sweater, their choice of clothes or all these put together!

Irrational feelings

Negative mindsets invariably produce irrational feelings about ourselves and these feelings often become self-fulfilling prophecies. For example, thinking 'I will never be any good with money' stops us trying to be good with money. 'I will never make anyone happy' stops us trying to make anyone happy and, concerning our ill health, 'I am no fun to have around any more' makes us stop trying to be good-humoured about the situation. These irrational feelings determine our behaviour. Unfortunately, chronic illness is often the spark that sets irrational feelings blazing out of control.

However, these feelings can be turned around. We can learn a new, more positive approach to life. First, however, we need to acknowledge our irrational thoughts and feelings for what they are, and for the behaviour they induce. Family celebrations commonly provoke feelings of anxiety in people with fibromyalgia. Actually writing down our negative thoughts and feelings, and really analysing them, can make the fact they are irrational crystal clear; it makes us more aware.

Here is an example of possible irrational thoughts and feelings prior to a family party.

Situation	Irrational thoughts	Irrational feelings
Family party	'I will be a real wet blanket. No one will want to talk to me. I will put a dampener on the whole event.'	'I will then feel sad, hurt and alienated. I will hate myself for being such a misery.'

This example illustrates just how irrational chronic illness can, at times, make us. Yet, if we do not analyse them, the potential repercussions can be staggering. In the example above, you may end up talking yourself into staying at home, experiencing a mixture of self-pity, guilt and even self-loathing. Your decision could even cause an argument with your partner ...

The example also reveals a common tendency for people to worry about something that may never happen. If it is Wednesday and you are in the middle of a flare-up, don't fret about a party scheduled for the weekend! You are hardly likely to be well enough to attend and your family should be made aware of that fact. However, if you are no worse than usual, then, realistically, staying at home is hardly the answer. No matter how dire your 'normal' condition, you need, for the sake of sanity, to have a life; you need to be with others occasionally, so you need to make an extra effort every now and again. Given sufficient forward planning, certain events really can be managed effectively. Whether your symptoms are severe or not, backing out of events/activities you may have enjoyed can leave you feeling angry with yourself, furious with your illness and resentful that everyone else is in good health!

I was taught to record my thoughts and feelings prior to a troublesome event and doing so always helps me. Try it and see if it helps you, too. Assuming, then, that you are no worse than usual, try to write down your assumptions about your presence at the party (as described in the example above). Now look objectively at what you have written. Are your thoughts and feelings reasonable? No doubt you would feel like a wet blanket if you sat with a face as long as a fiddle and made no effort to talk to anyone! Could you really be so rude that you would avoid talking with people? Are your relatives really so antisocial that they would disregard you?

When we challenge negative feelings in such a way, the reality of the situation soon becomes apparent. People make an effort to be friendly at family gatherings. Your fellow guests are people you know well. Common ground can always be found, should you wish to look for it.

So, you have re-evaluated and subsequently banished one set of negative thoughts, only to find it is swiftly replaced by another. You have decided to attend the party, but now you are worrying about coping with pain in company. Will the pain totally consume you? Will you burst into tears? Will everyone think you pathetic?

Although it is normal to worry about coping with pain when you are out of your usual environment, your worries may, due to your fears, be somewhat distorted. Writing them down helps you see them in a more detached light. Below, I have expanded on the example above by incorporating a column listing possible solutions.

Situation	Irrational thoughts	Irrational feelings	Solution
'I will be in a lot of pain at the party.'	'I will be unable to cope with the pain. I will feel as if I could cry. I will get angry and accuse everyone of not caring.'	'People will think me weak and stupid. They will hate me for spoiling the occasion. I will then feel angry with myself.'	'I will take painkillers before leaving and take more with me for later. I'll ask to lie down if I start to feel bad.'

Here, irrational feelings are seen for what they are and possible solutions are considered. Other solutions may include choosing the most supportive chair there, asking for a hot water bottle for your back or explaining in advance that you may have to leave early. After all, looking for realistic ways in which to ease a difficult situation is far more helpful than immersing yourself in worries that get you nowhere. More importantly, it can help you cope with some degree of pain.

You may then find yourself assailed by further worries. You have planned to ask if you may lie down, but, when the time comes, you feel anxious about actually doing so. Surely your hosts will think you feeble and demanding. Surely everyone will stare and whisper behind your back. This again is irrational thinking and as, obviously, you won't always be able to write your feelings down, you should mentally consider what you need to do. In this instance, all you can do – unless you want to risk incurring the usual thoughts of self-loathing and self-pity, on top of a certain increase in pain – is ask.

From personal experience, I can honestly say that people are only too willing to assist when asked directly. Often they haven't been sure what to say, but when you ask for help, it takes the pressure off them. They will likely then want to know whether the bedroom is warm enough, the bed firm enough, the pillows soft enough ... If they do scowl and make a comment to the effect that you are making a fuss – and in all my years of asking others for help regarding my fibromyalgia, I have never come across anyone who has – it says a lot more about their nature than yours!

Helping others to understand

In attempting to help the people you care about to understand your fibromyalgia, you should try to speak clearly and openly. Brevity also has a positive impact, as has being honest about how you feel.

Speaking openly

Before endeavouring to describe your feelings, you first need to focus on how you actually do feel. It may be difficult to admit you feel guilty, frustrated, angry, useless, vulnerable ... even to yourself. Sharing your feelings with others is even more difficult, yet it is an important step towards halting the problems those feelings can cause. In your need to be understood by others, however, you should be wary of making assumptions about how they feel about you.

Speaking to others in the following way is sure to cause offence: 'I get so upset when you think I'm exaggerating' or 'I don't believe you really care about me and that makes me feel so hopeless' or 'I'm losing confidence because you treat me as if I'm not trying to help myself.' Such comments will likely be seen as accusations; they may even provoke a quarrel. Speaking directly of your 'emotional problems' – without implying that the other person is contributing to those problems – will incline that person to take your comments more seriously. It should also encourage him or her to be more thoughtful in future. Before undertaking to speak openly of your feelings, however, the following list of considerations should be taken into account.

- *Ensure you have interpreted the other person's behaviour correctly.* For example, you may view your mother bringing you a basket of fruit and vegetables as a criticism of your diet when, in truth, it is a goodwill gesture, just to show she cares! You have a perfect right to interpret the words or actions of others in whatever way you wish, but that interpretation is not necessarily reality. In fact, it is amazing how wrong we often are in our perceptions of what others think and feel.

- *Ensure you are specific in recalling another person's behaviour.* For example, 'You never understand how exhausted I get', is far more inflammatory than 'You didn't seem to understand yesterday, when I told you how exhausted I felt.'
- *Ensure that what you are about to say is what you really mean.* For example, statements such as, 'Everyone thinks you're insensitive', 'We all think you've got an attitude problem' are, besides being inflammatory, very unfair. We have no way of knowing that 'everyone' is of the same opinion. The use of the depersonalized 'everyone', 'we' or 'us' – often said in the hope of deflecting the listener's anger – can cause more hurt and anger than if the criticism was direct and personal.

It's easy to see how others can misunderstand or take offence when we fail to communicate effectively. However, changing the habits of a lifetime is difficult. It means analysing our thoughts before rearranging them into speech. We are rewarded for our efforts, however, when people start to listen, when they cease to be annoyed as we carefully explain an area they don't fully understand. Once we have stopped trying to improve others, we can begin to focus on improving ourselves and our own situations.

Dealing with your co-workers

If you are managing to work and cope with fibromyalgia at the same time, well done! Exceptions for chronic ill health in the workplace generally have to be fought for. Even when your boss is tolerant, your co-workers often are not.

If your fibromyalgia is not yet acknowledged at work, be prepared for a struggle, but never be tempted to cover up your health-related shortcomings. Those who do so are rarely shown leniency. In fact, unless you are able to communicate the nature of your illness and how it affects your performance, you are liable to be condemned as slow and inefficient – especially by co-workers who are convinced you are not pulling your weight.

Strangely enough, given sufficient information about the illness, employers can be more sympathetic than some fellow employees. Your exclusion from certain duties can prompt certain co-workers to make snide remarks. Whether these remarks are related to jealousy, resentment, distrust or simply because you are an easy target when they are having a bad day, they are cruel and unjust, so should not be tolerated!

The thought of objecting to an unfair accusation, particularly when you are at a low ebb, may seem daunting. However, as well as being the only means of getting through to some people, it also helps you maintain your self-esteem. For example, a co-worker may remark, 'You look fine. I'm sure you're using your illness to get out of doing the filing!' Whether the tone is lighthearted or not, the content is hostile and undeserved. Failing to respond – maybe because you are too angry, too hurt, or simply too tired – only serves to confirm that opinion. Your answer should be a firm, 'I resent that. I'm glad you think I look OK, but I don't use my illness as an excuse, and I don't have to prove myself to you.' The co-worker will usually apologize at this point and may even confess, 'I suppose I just don't understand your illness.' Here is your chance to explain more about fibromyalgia.

Whenever others appear to be in a receptive frame of mind, try to grasp the opportunity to explain your condition. Your symptoms may best be understood when you equate them to something within the listener's experience. For instance, 'The fatigue can feel like the flu' or, to someone who has suffered sports injuries, 'The pain in my shoulder is like that of a torn ligament', helps that person see exactly how it is for you. Descriptive analogies can be effective, too (so long as you don't go over the top) – for example, 'The pain is like needles piercing the base of my neck', 'It feels like my back's been pummelled by a boxer', make the listener really think. Explain, too, the most troublesome of the additional symptoms from which you suffer, making sure to emphasize that they are all elements of your fibromyalgia. The more information you can feed to the people around you, the more likely they are to digest it.

Remember, too, that we should not expect everyone we encounter to be openly friendly, just as we may not be openly friendly towards everyone we meet. Some personalities just don't mix. Only in accepting this fact can you help yourself disregard those who refuse to listen.

Getting the best from your doctor

You may have suffered alarming symptoms for several months, expecting them to subside any day, but, instead, the mysteriously shifting pain persists, the headaches and fatigue have worsened and you have become sensitive to certain foods, certain chemicals, cold, damp and light. Feeling let down and confused when sympathetic ears become difficult to find, you turn to your doctor. You crave answers, but you worry that the doctor, like your family and friends, will think you are imagining it all. It is upsetting when people close to you are distrustful, but professional distrust is devastating.

Doctors are frequently baffled by the unusual symptoms of fibromyalgia and misdiagnosis – maybe one of anxiety, stress, depression, hysteria or some kind of neurosis – is not unusual. The misdiagnosis may be confirmed in your doctor's mind when you reply to the questions: 'Would you say you're a worrier?', 'How are you and your partner getting on?', 'Are you happy at work?' with a 'Since the illness took hold, I have been eaten up with worry, suffered relationship problems and had difficulties performing at work/getting along with co-workers.' The outcome may be a course of antidepressants, plus advice to the effect that you need a break from routine.

Few people with fibromyalgia have not had difficult dealings with doctors somewhere along the line. Yet, if your relationship with your doctor is not good, your health can suffer unnecessarily.

Poor communication on the part of the patient may, in the first place, lead to misdiagnosis. The following are examples of what can go wrong.

- For fear of being prejudged, patients tend to censor their descriptions of certain symptoms, such as anxiety, depression and so on.
- In their desperation to secure a diagnosis, patients may bombard – and therefore confuse – the doctor with a multitude of outwardly unrelated symptoms.
- In deference to the doctor's lack of time, patients may describe only their main symptom(s), omitting those that may otherwise help the doctor to arrive at an accurate conclusion.
- Keen to emphasize that they are neither lazy nor malingering, patients may incorrectly interpret the doctor's questions. For example, if the question 'How are your stamina levels?' comes

up, the patient may declare, 'I've never been one for sitting around. I've always had an active life.' The patient thereby frustrates the doctor's attempts to draw a clearer picture.

In order to secure a prompt and accurate diagnosis, you must:

- give your doctor a full and precise description of your symptoms;
- be sure you have understood the questions before replying;
- take care to speak clearly.

Moreover, try not to forget that doctors can only work within the confines of what they have been taught – evaluating symptoms in a scientific manner and looking to specific disorders as a result of your answers to the questions. Finally, I know it's difficult, but try not to expect immediate answers.

Remember, too, that your doctor is only human. Your 'attitude' may sway the conclusion arrived at. For example, if you are apologetic, the doctor may think you are imagining some of your symptoms. If you are angry with the doctor, the doctor may, in return, feel hurt and/or irritated.

As there is always the risk of a personality clash between a doctor and you, seek a doctor with whom you feel comfortable. Doctors have to maintain professional distance, but when you find one who is open-minded and understanding, hang on to him or her!

Adjusting your expectations

Thinking about the future is a natural human characteristic. We enjoy looking forward to holidays and certain other forthcoming events; we need to look ahead and project possible outcomes before we can make any kind of decision. However, when that future is clouded by the pain and fear that comes with chronic illness, we are plagued by compelling 'What if ...' questions. The bleak and hopeless years we visualize as our future appear beyond our control, yet they can haunt our waking hours as well as our dreams.

Pain will always induce anxiety, as it is hard not to fear a pain-filled future. However, looking ahead in fear is counter-productive. The first step towards conquering the inclination to worry about what may or may not happen is to tell yourself that it does no good. Controlling your thinking is far from easy, but it can be achieved. When the bleak visions loom, try to distract yourself either by turning your mind to something pleasant or, fibromyalgia withstanding, doing something requiring concentration. After such 'visions' have been staved off on a regular basis, the propensity towards that type of thinking will gradually decrease.

Living in the present

People with fibromyalgia need all their resources to handle the present. A calm and contented now is more emotionally nourishing than a mind reeling with the upsets the future may or may not hold. In the same way, cherishing the moment is preferable to letting it slip by unappreciated because we are too busy thinking ahead. How many of us look forward to seeing a film, a band, recital, play, but don't think to enjoy the journey there? How many of us look forward to summer, forgetting to appreciate spring? It is the same with numerous things in our lives.

'However,' you may ask, 'is it possible for people with chronic pain to master the art of living in the present?' As people with fibromyalgia have, of necessity, to always remember to pace themselves, finding enjoyable yet untaxing leisure interests is essential. After all, why sit brooding when you could be reading a gripping book, penning a poem, surfing the Internet, taking a walk or sharing views with someone close? This is the time to consider doing things you never had time for before. If, for example, assembling a model railway was a childhood dream you never managed to fulfil or if you always fancied learning to play the piano, but never quite got around to it, this, fibromyalgia permitting, is your opportunity!

Making the most of now

When you need to rest all day in anticipation of an evening out, it is important that you enjoy the day as well. OK, so you dare not risk tackling housework, neither dare you go into town, but there is sure to be something agreeable with which you can occupy yourself in the meantime. This is your chance to select that new jacket from your catalogue, update your stamp collection, muse over last year's holiday photos or simply watch that new comedy DVD.

Those of you who dare not risk even sitting during the intervening hours may find lying on the sofa to read, watching TV or listening to music an acceptable alternative. At times, I need to spend several hours a day lying on my back in bed, which means that, until my husband and I can afford to reinforce the bedroom ceiling, I am unable to even watch TV. Believe me, having little to do but listen to music for hours made me feel very sorry for myself – that is, until I discovered audio books. Most libraries stock a varied selection, mostly comprising bestsellers, and, for a small fee, will loan up to six 'books' at a time. People receiving benefits are entitled to a free ticket. Give them a try. They may broaden your life, as they have mine!

Looking on the bright side

Developing a positive outlook is invaluable in fibromyalgia. It stops us from dwelling on the past, helps us to enjoy the present and bestows hope and conviction. When we look for something pleasing in the things we do – even chores – we can significantly lighten our load.

You may be wondering, 'What could possibly be pleasing about washing dishes or peeling potatoes?' As most of us perform these tasks by the kitchen window, they have that in their favour. While you scour the pans or wash or peel the spuds, do you consciously appreciate the world outside or are you inclined to gaze blindly out, fretting about this and that? If the latter is generally the case, try to concentrate instead on really looking at, and appreciating, your outdoor environment. Admire the manifold creations of nature, observe the inventiveness in all that is made by human hands, notice how people behave as they go about their daily business.

As the seasons pass, consciously appreciate the effects different weather conditions have on your environment. Even the busiest and most depressing of streets can be enhanced by bright sunshine sparkling on wet rooftops, mist gliding in graceful ribbons through the air, glassy icicles hanging from window ledges, a covering of fresh snow. Enhanced? When you need to hire a JCB (and an operator) to clear pathways through the snow? When it's so foggy you need a searchlight to find the front gate? When it's so slippery you need spikes on your shoes?

All right, so 'inclement' weather can create numerous problems, but why think of those problems when you're snug and warm indoors? Keep your mind on the present. Let gazing at the weather – the rain, the frost, the snow – stir your senses. Children like to stretch out a hand to feel the rain, they are awed by the sight of icicles and they are so excited by snow. Often we lose that childish appreciation when we reach adulthood, but it's never too late to recapture it! The time to worry about harsh weather conditions is only shortly before you step outside!

Accepting what you can't change

Including the weather, there are many things in life we cannot change. We can do nothing about the fact that we are either creative or practical, black or white, tall or short (or anything in between). Neither can we change the fact that we have fibromyalgia, although we can certainly improve the situation. However, acknowledging what we can't change, and trying to live with it, is fundamental to stress management. In accepting things as they stand, we say goodbye to a great deal of frustration.

Keeping to the weather analogy a while longer, it has to be said that some of us have little choice, after assessing the situation rationally, but to virtually hibernate during a prolonged cold spell. Sadly, despite the fact that feeling distanced from the rest of the world is profoundly disheartening, you can do nothing about harsh weather.

In fine weather, and barring flare-ups, you may find it easier to get out and about. You may need help with the shopping, someone with you when you visit the museum, library, hairdresser or car boot sale, but you should make the most of being able to do these things. Winter, in particular, is the time to consider taking up new interests, to think about doing things you never got round to before.

As well as being distracting, involving yourself in a new challenge can be infinitely rewarding. Consider playing computer games, talking to others with fibromyalgia via the Internet, taking up model making, woodwork, metal work, oil painting, stencilling, photography, playing the keyboard, tapestry work, glass and china painting, picture framing, jewellery making ... the list is endless. The selection of 'things to do' in a craft shop alone is quite dazzling!

Of course, not everyone with fibromyalgia is physically able to do these things. They are merely suggestions. People who have difficulty leaning forward may be unable to sketch, paint, sew or make models; people who are unable to tilt their heads are similarly limited, as are those who are physically incapable of holding out an arm for a period of time. The challenge is to find interests to suit your capabilities, as well as ones that stimulate your imagination.

Learning to let go

When fibromyalgia takes hold, many of us have no alternative but to relinquish a lifetime's ambitions. We give up our careers, then, as a consequence, feel we have lost much of what gave us a sense of worth and identity. However, learning to let go of what we can no longer do – possibly looking to a new, less ambitious but equally fulfilling career and searching out new interests to replace old ones – is the only way forward emotionally. People with fibromyalgia need to look after their minds as well as their bodies.

If you have had to give up your job, studying part-time at your local college will help you feel less isolated. Whether you fancy acquiring a few academic qualifications or simply want to take up a new leisure interest (where the atmosphere is more casual and regular attendance not so important), learning something different can be rewarding. Studying a subject that is helpful in dealing with fibromyalgia – homeopathy, reflexology, aromatherapy, meditation, relaxation, stress management or assertiveness training, say – may prove invaluable, too.

CLAIT (computer literacy and information technology) courses can be useful if you are either looking for a new career, want to use a computer for your own purposes or are hoping to work from home. A college prospectus can be obtained from your local library or council information office. Where vocational courses are concerned, people receiving state benefits may not have to pay tuition fees. Your college welfare officer will be able to give you full details. It is important that you inform your tutor of your fibromyalgia-related limitations at the outset. Allowances will then be made if you are slow to produce work, time off will be understood and you may even be given the most comfortable chair!

If you are fairly mobile, aqua-aerobics, low-impact aerobics and/or yoga classes can, if you employ caution, be beneficial. Such 'training' should not only help maintain and ultimately improve your strength, stamina and mobility, it can also provide an outlet for stress. Competitive games – even those of a gentle nature, such as chess, backgammon, roulette, bridge – are not a good idea. They produce tension and stress and, if you lose the game, feelings of uselessness and despair.

Perhaps you have already found that fibromyalgia itself can be the gateway to a whole new field of opportunity. Fibromyalgia support groups are springing up all over the UK, each of which needs ongoing assistance of one kind or another. Practical help at group meetings and fundraising events is always required. If you are not physically able to stand at a tombola or 'nearly new' stall or make and distribute cups of tea at an open-day meeting, you may be able to assist by contributing to the group's newsletter, donating articles/tea and biscuits for the next table-top sale, providing ideas for fundraising or offering suggestions for 'speakers'.

In fact, if you would like to involve yourself further in the group's activities, you could offer to become a committee member. People who participate in voluntary work invariably report a rise in their self-esteem. If your particular talent is handling money, you could offer to be treasurer; if you have clerical experience, you could volunteer to be secretary; if you are good at organizing or dealing with people, you could be social secretary or, if you enjoy writing, you could edit the newsletters. If you possess people skills, common sense as well as a management background (although this is not essential), maybe you could even think of setting up and chairing a support group of your own. There are still many areas not catered for by existing groups.

Smile for a while

'All things are cause either for laughter or weeping,' wrote Seneca, the Roman philosopher. It is true that comedy and tragedy are close bedfellows, for both are reflex actions rooted in the central nervous system and its related hormones.

How we respond to a certain stimulus depends on our outlook on life. Letting go of the past and our fears for the future is 'releasing'. It allows us to smile more. The saying that 'laughter is the best medicine' is particularly true for chronic pain patients. Laughter is also the most difficult emotional response to achieve when we are in pain. However, the people who manage to smile a lot, who manage to see the lighter side of different situations, deal more effectively with their pain. Fibromyalgia is not a funny condition – it causes a lot of grief and disability – yet a surprising number of people retain (or evolve) a good sense of humour.

Laughing at yourself in particular can be more therapeutic than a whole-body massage, it can be more releasing than sex or alcohol and it invariably makes other people warm to you. When you laugh, your muscles relax, bleak thoughts lift and 'feel-good' endorphins are released into your bloodstream. As a result, you feel uplifted and bright!

Adjusting your lifestyle

On a more practical level, it is vital that people with fibromyalgia focus on all they do in the course of a day. Only by being constantly aware can you avoid unnecessary pain. Being conscious of the way you dress, sit and perform tasks requires a lot of effort, but can become second nature once you have learned to adjust behaviours identified as pain-provoking and reaped the benefits of doing this.

Identifying problems

As low muscle endurance causes numerous problems in fibro-myalgia, try to always assess the possible repercussions before going ahead with any activity. Consider first the way you move. How do you get out of bed? Do you sit bolt upright, then clumsily climb out, or do you ease yourself to the edge, then carefully 'roll' out? How do you shower? Do you scrub yourself vigorously or do you soap/sponge yourself carefully? How do you dress? Do you hop around on one leg as you struggle into your tights/trousers or do you sit down and carefully pull them on?

The operative word is 'carefully'. If you think yourself through your daily routine, you will likely find many examples of where the word 'carefully' should be – but is not – applied. But 'care' is perhaps your greatest weapon. Use it and you can prevent the muscle damage that leads to a full-scale flare-up, as well as the myriad of emotional problems tied into any exacerbation of symptoms.

Next, you should evaluate the way you perform tasks around the house. Housework has many pitfalls for someone with fibromy-algia. Vacuuming is off limits for most people with the condition, as is lifting furniture, decorating and heavy cleaning. Jobs such as cooking, baking, washing, ironing and shopping carry a high risk for some people with fibromyalgia and the possible repercussions should be considered carefully before going ahead.

If, for example, moving the sofa to clean behind it instigated a previous flare-up, ask yourself whether you really want a repeat performance. Try to learn from your experiences. Look for and examine possible solutions. Cooking, for instance, can be made easier by buying occasional microwave meals, frozen vegetables and takeaway food. Show family members how grateful you are when they prepare a meal in advance and they may offer to do it regularly! However, lifting heavy pans off the hob and trays/dishes out of the oven is, for many with fibromyalga, too risky. The solution may be in timing the meal so that a family member can, on arriving home from work, dish it up. If you are in no condition even to attempt cooking, you must find some way of passing the task to someone else. The key is to know your limitations and to abide by them.

Other housework – dusting, washing-up, wiping kitchen surfaces, cleaning the bathroom and hanging out washing – can seem too simple to even think of giving up. However, consider for a moment the demands these activities exert on your energy-depleted, pain-disposed body. For a start, although dusting is viewed as a light task, it demands excesses of movement. You may need to kneel or bend to dust the fire-surround, you may need to stretch to dust the wall unit or bookshelves, you may need to lean over the TV to dust the window ledge. See what I mean? When you wash up, you stand still, often in a slightly hunched position, and scouring pans and baking trays requires you to exert a surprising amount of pressure. Wiping kitchen surfaces makes you tense, stoop and use pressure; cleaning the bathroom requires that you bend, stretch and use pressure; and hanging out washing involves bending, lifting and stretching!

All these movements can cause your pain levels to rise. If, after considering the possible consequences, you feel you can perform a task without there being a pay-back later, still use caution. Lifting anything moderately heavy is not wise. If you are fairly confident that you can lift, say, a wet sheet from the laundry basket, ensure that your back, hips and head are correctly aligned. When you need to use pressure, say when polishing or ironing, keep your body as relaxed as possible and take regular breaks. If you feel the slightest elevation of your normal levels of discomfort, rest immediately. There is always another day.

Re-evaluating non-essential activities

There are perhaps several activities that, although you know them to be risky, you nevertheless continue to perform. You would be well advised to regularly review their importance, however. For instance, you may unwittingly be aggravating your condition by washing your hair every morning in winter. If this is the case, ask yourself if it is crucial, now that temperatures have fallen and you're feeling delicate, that you do so. Wouldn't washing it once or twice a week be sufficient? Could you even consider having your hair restyled for the duration of winter? Easy-to-manage hairstyles are not necessarily unflattering!

Other 'necessary' activities should be regularly assessed, too. For example, is it imperative that you dust the living room every day? Wouldn't once or twice a week be adequate here, too? Do underwear, tea towels and so on desperately need ironing? Surely a few crumples in such items can be overlooked? Do you have to haul shopping all the way from the supermarket? Shopping via the Internet or by phone to supermarkets that deliver the goods to your home at a time convenient to you is now available. If this facility is not yet operating in your area, consider returning with your shopping by taxi or, better still, get someone else to do it!

Depending on your present state of health, you could also ask yourself whether or not it is important that you do all the washing-up. Wouldn't it be safer, if you are feeling fragile, to leave the dishes in water for someone else to deal with later? Do you have to go out to pay bills when you're really not up to it? Wouldn't it be easier to set up 'direct debits' from your bank account? Should you really be trailing around town looking for household items when your legs are painful already? Wouldn't it be better to order them from a catalogue?

Heeding past pain triggers

Fibromyalgia is a frustrating business, not least because the boundaries of what we can and cannot do are continually shifting. Delayed pain, arising from the low muscle stamina situation affecting all people with fibromyalgia, means that a task we accomplish with little pay-back one week can give rise to a full-scale flare-up the next. This factor is then complicated by a sensitivity to cold, heat, stress and so on. It is essential, therefore, that we learn from our experiences, taking account of all problem areas.

We are often at our lowest physical and emotional ebb during the early months/years of the illness, when, loath to abandon the activities that afford us a sense of 'self', purpose and worth, we are inclined to ignore past pain triggers. We are afraid of 'giving in' to the illness, fearing that if we stop pushing ourselves, we may end up being incapable of anything. Only with the realization that such behaviour is actually aggravating the illness do we eventually change our ways. Uncertainty regarding exactly where our boundaries lie, however, can cause us to then go through a period of overprotecting ourselves.

There is nothing more disconcerting than knowing that, in undertaking almost any activity, there is a risk of inducing an increase in pain or a full symptom flare-up. However, the risk can be minimized by constant wariness, remembering to always pace yourself, keeping your body relaxed and moving cautiously. Unfortunately, it is not possible to *eliminate* risk in fibromyalgia. Effectively coming to a full stop would arrest feelings of achievement, reduce stamina and cause muscle wastage. You can only retain, and ultimately improve, the strength you have by being as active as possible – without overdoing it! It is important that you constantly strive, therefore, to achieve a balance between too much and too little activity. 'Easier said than done', I can almost hear you say and how right you are!

In order to achieve a balance – keeping in mind that the scales will keep tilting – you should consider past pain triggers. For example, if cleaning the car last month resulted in an exacerbation of pain, you should ask yourself these questions.

- Were you up to undertaking the task in the first place?
- Did you work just as quickly as before you got ill?
- Did you clean the whole car without pausing?
- Did you put on a spurt when your pain levels began rising?

A positive answer to any of the above would account for the extra pain! Now reassess the whole procedure. Wouldn't it be better, if you are well enough, to clean the bodywork on Monday morning, taking care to work slowly and carefully, then rest Monday afternoon? If there is no worsening of symptoms, maybe the windows could be cleaned on Tuesday and so on.

When, after due deliberation, you decide to tackle a certain task/activity, always attend to the way you go about it. Instead of proceeding with the vigour born of long years of habit, take care to work slowly and cautiously, with your body in a stable and balanced position. It is equally important that you stop what you are doing and rest as soon as you feel your normal pain levels rising. If you don't break off immediately, you may bring on a flare-up lasting weeks!

Being assertive

Trying always to please others, put others first, is counter-productive. Rather than inspiring admiration, pushing yourself beyond your limits makes others suppose that you are doing what you are capable of doing. They will expect the same from you every time. Avoid risking extra pain and maintain your self-respect by learning, instead, to please yourself. Try, too, to speak up when you need a helping hand.

Asking for help is not easy, especially when you have been active and independent all your life. Yet communicating your needs will usually get you what you want. What is the alternative? – frustration and anger. Asking for help is not an indication of weakness or failure. It is a sign of your resolve to face your situation, to be less of an emotional drain on the people around you. Rather than have you angry because he or she is unable to anticipate your needs, your partner or friend would surely prefer that you speak out.

There is a fine line between being assertive and being demanding, however! Asking for help clearly and politely, then showing gratitude afterwards creates 'feel-good' emotions in others. It also increases the chances of their offering help in the future.

Encouraging flexibility in the people around you is important, too. It can reduce the pressure to 'oblige'. For example, preparing friends for a possible last-minute cancellation on your part minimizes their disappointment – and your resulting guilt – if you do have to cancel. Likewise, warning co-workers that you may not be up to finishing that piece of work over the weekend prepares them for the possibility of having to do it on Monday.

Learning to say 'no'

Saying 'no' to others is equally difficult but, for the sake of your health, you need to say it, and as often as necessary. Again, until told otherwise, the people in your life will simply assume you are still able to do most things.

If, after friends 'expect' you to drive 20 miles to visit them, help them move house or babysit their toddler, your pleas of ill health are disregarded, your safest option is to say a definite 'no'. Go on to illustrate exactly why you are refusing.

Taking the first example, you could explain, 'If I drove over to you, I'd not be up to much else. It's been a while since we met and I was looking forward to a good chat.' Your friends will likely admit they didn't realize how ill you were and offer to drive to your home instead. However, if they are not satisfied with your reasoning, you should dig in your heels and add, 'Then the drive home would be a nightmare. To be honest, I'd be in so much pain I wouldn't be safe behind the wheel! I'd be grateful if you could come to see me instead.' If these people are worthy of the title 'friends', they will now readily agree to your suggestion.

To the friends who expect you to help them move house, you could say, 'I'm sorry, but I can't. If I tried lifting furniture I'd end up rigid with pain – and I'm not exaggerating.' If they have helped you a lot in the past, you could add, 'I'll be happy to bring you a casserole/stand you a takeaway for tea, though.' The response will probably be sympathy for your ill health, together with gratitude for offering alternative assistance.

To the friends who have asked you to babysit their toddler, you could say, 'I'd love to look after little Katy, but I'm just not well enough. What most concerns me is that I wouldn't be able to leap up if she was about to hurt herself.' Wanting the best for their daughter, your friends would probably say a hurried, 'Oh, I see. Don't worry, we'll get so-and-so to look after her!'

Don't, in any circumstance, allow anyone to pressure you into doing something you know will provoke pain. Also, don't put yourself under pressure by feeling obliged to repay someone in kind. Your health is far more important than feelings of duty.

The people around you

People with fibromyalgia desperately need to know that others care. Most of all they crave the sympathy and understanding of their nearest and dearest, feeling upset when they are shown thought-lessness or impatience. Yet those with the condition often fail to appreciate that the illness can create huge problems for these very people.

Fibromyalgia and your partner

Our partners – on whom we tend to rely most for emotional support – are often more troubled by our ill health than we realize. They can feel guilty for being well and active when we are sick and stagnant, disappointed and confused when we show no sign of recovery, angry and useless for seeming never to be able to say the right thing and, not least, anxious for their own future happiness.

In fact, our partners' concerns are possibly equal to our own. Their need for intimacy, companionship and a future they can look forward to – mixed with feelings of inadequacy for being unable to ease our suffering – may even prompt doubts about their ability to cope indefinitely with a partner who is chronically ill. Their misgivings can then be amplified when they endure endless reproaches for being insensitive and uncaring.

A person who is chronically ill can become self-absorbed. The main causes of this are that:

- the physical and emotional drain of dealing with the condition can interfere with the person's ability to see his or her partner's viewpoint;
- and/or after experiencing little but scepticism or indifference from others, the person may misinterpret his or her partner's behaviour as more of the same.

When a communication breakdown occurs, the relationship can become a battle, with each partner feeling resentful and unloved. Unless each makes an effort to understand the other person, the relationship may flounder. It is a fact that you can only know what your partner is thinking and feeling when you make time to calmly talk problems through. It is certainly worth the effort for exchanging perceptions, fears and needs carries the bonus of strengthening your relationship.

Fibromyalgia and other family members

Just as your partner has his or her own needs, so too have other family members. Their needs are essentially selfish, as are everyone's. In most cases, their chief need, where you are concerned, is to see you well and smiling again. They won't then have to worry about you so much, they won't then be obliged to be so attentive. Once you are 'recovered', you will again be able to accompany them on Saturday shopping sessions, go to line dancing class or play snooker and squash ... Put simply, you are an important part of their lives and they want everything to be back to normal.

As your illness continues, however, their bafflement may turn to irritation. Desperate to see you well, they may prefer to interpret your behaviour as lethargy, self-indulgence or hypochondria rather than true chronic illness. Remarks such as, 'You're not doing anything to help yourself', 'You need to get out and enjoy yourself more' are typical, made in the misguided belief that you need a 'push' to help you back to 'normality'.

Unchecked, such 'advice' can turn to full-scale nagging. Comments such as, 'You should try running up and down the stairs 20 times a day – that'll improve your stamina', 'Get out on your bicycle again. It'll do you the power of good', 'Are you sure you're trying hard enough? Don't you want to get better?' may be delivered repeatedly in a genuine desire to see you fit and well, but they are hurtful and demoralizing. When told often enough that you are making no effort to improve your condition, you can start to believe it.

Ironically, the people closest to us are the ones most likely to make damaging remarks, which in fact only compounds our hurt. However, we should try to remember that they are the people who are most concerned that we get better. Instead of observing the situation from all angles, they make the mistake of seeing it through their eyes only.

Daniel and Helen

It is easy to understand why 10-year-old Daniel has convinced himself that his mother, Helen, 39, is not so ill as she says she is. He needs her to make his meals, run him around in the car, organize his life ... just to be there as her normal, capable self. He sees her illness as a threat to his whole world. She *looks* fine – just the same as ever. In attempting to prove to himself that everything is indeed exactly as it always was,

Daniel will often say, 'You look fine, Mum. Take me to my friend's house tonight, will you?' When Helen, feeling guilty, explains that she's not up to driving the car, Daniel bursts out, 'You don't want to do anything for me any more! I don't think you love me!' So, despite the fact that Helen is in pain, she gets into the car and takes her son to see his friend. Consequently, Daniel is reassured, but Helen, in more pain than ever, is upset that her child can't seem to understand.

Daniel's demands persist because, in capitulating, Helen is proving she can still do as much as ever for him. He will only accept her illness if she continually reassures him of her love, yet firmly explains why she cannot be as active as before. When children know where they stand, they soon adapt.

Sarah and Michael

Sarah, 30, is mother to 18-month-old Bethany and has recently been diagnosed as having fibromyalgia. She makes keeping Bethany clean, safe and fed a priority, but feels a failure for neglecting the housework, annoyed that her husband, Michael, expects home life to be as happy and ordered as it was before she became ill, and cheated for being too ill to *enjoy* Bethany.

Their respective parents occasionally offer to babysit, but Sarah invariably feels too ill to go out. This is yet another bone of contention between Michael and herself.

People with fibromyalgia who have young children need a lot of practical help and need to do a lot of straight talking to relatives and friends. Sarah cannot, realistically, be expected to care for a toddler all day, as well as perform all the other tasks in the home. She needs to calmly inform Michael, their families and close friends exactly how ill and miserable she feels, making it clear that, as well as daily help, she needs rest periods and quality time with her child. If no one volunteers assistance (people usually do offer to help at this point), she will need to ask for it outright. She and Michael should then ask family and friends to have Bethany at weekends – maybe draw up a rota. As she nears nursery age, Social Services may step in to arrange early entry into nursery school.

Peter and his parents

Joan and Derek are the parents of Peter, who is 48, married, and has two sons. Peter has fibromyalgia. Joan and Derek have always enjoyed holidays with Peter and his family, but they now feel these are in jeopardy. They had proudly watched Peter's career, which he has suddenly abandoned, and they had hoped to rely on him a bit more as they grew older. In addition, they had formerly felt a sense of satisfaction at seeing him happy with his life. Observing that he is now unhappy and in pain has even induced feelings of failure in them. Many parents measure their parenting success by the health, happiness and prosperity of their children.

Finding it difficult to cope with Peter's anguish, unwilling to accept that he is as incapacitated as he says he is, they constantly compare 'then' with 'now'. They see a man who has lost his 'status' in life, whose wife and children are increasingly unhappy and, because he is no longer able to provide, is struggling financially. They make comparisons with how active and alert they were at his age, how they enjoyed family life and how they managed to care for their own ageing parents.

As Peter shows no signs of recovery, Joan and Derek's scepticism increases. They convince themselves that if he 'pulls himself together' he will quickly return to normal. As more time elapses, they decide that his illness is imaginary, preferring to think he is suffering from mental instability than from fibromyalgia – a condition of which, after all, they have never heard.

Peter needs to sit down with his parents and firmly assert that their attitude is hurting him. Seen, for the first time, from their son's viewpoint, they will probably realize that their behaviour has indeed been inappropriate and may even apologize. This is Peter's opportunity to tell them more about the illness, backing up his words with literature on the subject. His parents may occasionally revert to the old misconceptions, but should be willing to re-evaluate their behaviour as and when it is pointed out.

Rebecca and her mother

Some family situations have become too fraught to simply be altered by a few firm words. Rebecca, 26, is resentful that 54-year-old Margaret, her fibromyalgic mother, is not there for her any more. She accuses Margaret of 'wallowing in self-pity' and 'demanding attention for an illness she hasn't got'. Margaret reacts angrily and the situation quickly spirals out of control. Rebecca may even refuse to let her children see their grandmother, declaring that as she is 'off her head', she would upset them. This state of events is profoundly disturbing to Margaret, for not only does she feel an incredible sense of loss (similar to that of being bereaved), she may also assume she is responsible for the rift.

Rather than trying to get through to her daughter, Margaret would be best advised to keep out of her life for a time. However, she must remember that she has done nothing wrong. She suffers from a debilitating illness, which should be received with an open mind. OK, so she lost her temper when Rebecca was mean, but that is understandable.

In waiting for Rebecca to calm down, she offers her daughter an opportunity to examine *her* behaviour.

If some time elapses and still Rebecca makes no contact, I would suggest that Margaret make the first move. She should say, 'I'm sorry things got so heated. I said some stupid things.' I anticipate that Rebecca will also apologize, allowing her mother to add, 'I have been very ill, and I get frustrated when you don't seem to understand. Can we talk about it some more?' If Rebecca again erects a brick wall, it is best to keep some distance between them. However, I expect that, at this juncture, Rebecca will make more of an effort to understand.

Coping with chronic pain

Pain is transmitted to the brain via two types of nerves, each working independently of the other, and each having a different structure. 'Fast pain' – that arising from a cut, toothache or broken limb – is quickly relayed to the central nervous system (CNS) located in the brain, but the actual pain is felt at the level of the tissues, often provoking a reflex action of instantly withdrawing from the pain source. In fast pain, the hurt can stop fairly rapidly, too.

'Deep pain', on the other hand, travels relatively slowly and the resulting pain sensations are felt at the level of the CNS. This type of pain lingers longer than that of fast pain, its transmissions normally associated with chronic pain conditions, such as fibromyalgia, rheumatoid arthritis and osteoarthritis. The 'spillover' of certain chemicals in the muscles in fibromyalgia further aggravates the situation, causing the sensation of pain to spread to nearby healthy tissues – in this instance perhaps travelling from the neck into the shoulders, back and face/jaw (see Chapter 1).

Although a small proportion of the pain of fibromyalgia is thought to be fast pain – felt at tissue level – the greater proportion is believed to be deep pain. Individuals with a deep pain problem are also far less likely to obtain relief from painkilling medication (narcotics and analgesics) than are those with a fast pain problem. However, new kinds of medication continue to emerge and medical professionals are becoming more open to using 'invasive' treatments for severe pain (see Chapter 3 for details of medications available at the time of writing).

Natural painkillers

On a more positive note, we also know that the body is capable of generating painkilling 'feel-good' neurotransmitters (endorphins and enkephalins) by natural means. Pleasurable activities, positive thinking, total relaxation and exercise (careful, non-taxing exercise where fibromyalgia is concerned) can all produce a satisfying 'high' or feelings of serenity. Both states actively block a degree of pain. Alternatively, negative thoughts and feelings, along with long-term inactivity and/or dependency on medication, can suppress the production of these 'feel-good' chemicals, thereby limiting the individual's ability to deal with pain.

Distraction

Living with chronic pain is a formidable affair. The awareness that we may never be entirely rid of it creates negative emotions that, if we fail to devise ways of managing the pain, can be overwhelming.

The simplest coping strategy is distraction – awareness of pain fades when the mind is pleasantly occupied. The intensity of any pain, however, can be greatly influenced by the situation in which it is experienced. Throughout history, there have been numerous accounts of soldiers fighting on despite terrible injuries, only becoming conscious of their pain when the battle was over. The theory that circumstances peculiar to each case are responsible for a variance in pain levels was supported by research in the 1950s, when it was found that wounded soldiers complained far less during recuperation than did civilians facing various types of surgery. The main difference was that the former had many dis-tractions from their pain. They felt relief at still being alive and knew that, for them, the battle was over and they would likely soon be returned to their families, all of which probably acted as a painkiller in itself. The civilians, on the other hand, had no such strong positive thoughts about their stay in hospital. Indeed, they were worried about spending time in alien surroundings, being away from their families and, not least, about the operation going wrong.

The distraction technique can easily be applied to our everyday lives. For example, engaging in cheery conversation, reading a light-hearted book, watching a comedy on TV, lovemaking or expe-riencing pleasing therapies, such as aromatherapy or reflexology, can occupy the senses and effectively reduce the awareness of pain. Indeed, finding pleasurable distractions can be one of our greatest allies in our quest to manage the pain.

However, beware! Due to the delayed response situation caused by low muscle endurance – the presence of which typifies fibro-myalgia – pain must never be entirely blocked from the conscious mind. Anticipation is your best weapon here. In the early stages of pain progression, stop and think what you need to do in order to intercept its course. In order to detect an early build-up of pain, constant, low-key awareness of your body is essential.

Staying active

When you feel constantly wiped out, when it seems that all you do causes pain, it may be tempting to take to your bed. Limited bed-rest is beneficial in a flare-up, but if you don't attempt to exercise on a fairly regular basis, your body can become stiff and less efficient, your limbs more painful and your muscles will likely waste.

Holding yourself stiffly encourages pain, as does limiting your-self from making specific movements. If, for example, your neck is painful when you move your head, trying to avoid doing so indefi-nitely will cause the muscles to become less flexible and enforced movement to become more painful. It's a catch-22 situation. You limit your head movements because they cause pain, then, because your neck muscles become weaker, the pain increases. The only answer – painful though it may be – is to begin gentle neck exercises.

Crisis medication

We live in a society that is over-reliant on drugs. A prescription for medication of some kind is expected of a visit to the doctor and self-medication is encouraged by media advertising. Painkillers, anti-inflammatory drugs and muscle relaxants are beneficial in the short term, but prolonged usage can produce side effects ranging from mild digestive problems to liver or kidney damage, as well as tolerance, which is when the patient needs to take more and more of a certain drug to achieve the same effect. Another side effect may be 'brain fog', the presence of which impedes the clear thinking often required to regain control over your life.

Medication can, however, reduce pain to a level at which gentle exercise can be resumed, thereby strengthening the tissues. In the early stages of illness, it can also help to reduce underlying tension. These benefits aside because, with time, their side effects often surpass their benefits, they are best used briefly. Long-term pain management can, therefore, be more successfully achieved by natural means.

Electrical stimulators (TENS)

Transcutaneous Electrical Nerve Stimulation (TENS) machines provide effective pain relief for many people, without the risk of side effects. The small, battery-operated devices, easily attached to the waistband of a skirt or trousers, transmit electrical impulses to electrodes that adhere to painful areas. The machine produces a tingling/pulsating sensation as it transmits electrical impulses to the CNS, thereby blocking sensations of pain.

In addition, electrical stimulation is believed to encourage the release of endorphins – the natural painkillers produced in the brain. TENS machines can be worn from early morning until bedtime, but up to one hour of usage may be required before benefit is felt.

The people who are lucky enough to experience relief from their TENS machines daily may be able to eliminate drugs entirely. However, many find that, although the treatment works well at first, it becomes less effective after a few weeks. This probably occurs because the CNS overrides the effects of repeated interference. Devices that overcome this problem by randomly switching stimulation on and off are currently being developed. In the meantime, using the machine for maybe two hours, then turning it off for two hours (or whatever timescale is relevant to your levels of pain) can prolong its usefulness.

Pain clinic patients may be allowed free use of a TENS machine. Alternatively, machines may be hired or purchased from certain chemists.

Improving sleep

Pain levels commonly rise when sleep is more disturbed than usual. Stress is often at the root of sleep disturbance, for there is nothing worse for mind and body than anxiously tossing and turning.

When stress can be relieved by a simple positive action, however, do it! For example, explaining to a friend that you aren't up to a particular activity or securing a promise of help with your weekend shopping should immediately put your mind at ease.

When stress arises due to a deep-seated concern – maybe you are worried that, because you are stumbling over your words more lately, your condition is deteriorating or perhaps you know your son is playing truant from school – the problem should again be resolved as soon as possible. In the first instance, you should see your doctor at the earliest opportunity. Hopefully, the doctor will quickly reassure you that a good relaxation strategy will effectively restore – or at least improve – your speech. (If you ask for details in this respect, the doctor will point you in the right direction.) In the second instance, you and your partner should talk with the child in order to discover the root of the problem. You should then devise with his teachers a stage 1 'rescue' plan. With any luck, you will soon be sleeping better.

Over-the-counter medications can increase the duration of sleep, but will not lengthen deep sleep, essential for the repair and regeneration of tissues. However, tricyclic antidepressants, available on prescription, can encourage deep sleep. If your prescribed medication is no longer effective, the dosage may need adjusting.

When pain prevents you from getting to sleep, try taking your usual painkillers at bedtime. If discomfort due to lying in one position for too long wakes you up, evaluate the comfort of your bed. Although a reasonably firm bed is recommended for people with fibromyalgia, you may find it helps to place a duvet between the mattress and sheet. The surface 'give' this offers is kind on sore muscles. Neck support in the form of a surgical collar (see your doctor about this) or a specially moulded pillow can be helpful, too. When lying on your back, place a pillow beneath your knees to take the strain off your lower back, hips and legs.

Develop good sleep habits by doing the following:

- unwind before going to bed by listening to music or a relaxation tape, reading or watching an unemotive programme on TV;
- have a warm drink;
- shortly before bedtime, take a warm bath (preferably using relaxing aromatherapy oils – see page 91);

- go to bed as soon as you feel sleepy – don't wait up until your usual bedtime;
- ensure that your bed and bedroom are warm;
- once in bed, breathe slowly and evenly, not shallowly, but using your diaphragm (see page 156), clear your mind and allow your thoughts to drift – don't hold on to any one thought, let each pass unchecked;
- get up at the same time every morning.

Try to avoid the following:

- caffeine drinks after 6 p.m.;
- engaging in animated conversation (or arguments) before bedtime;
- napping during the day;
- sitting watching TV for long periods, particularly in the evening.

Taking up the last point, sitting to watch TV for several hours during daytime and evening is, for many of us, a habit that not only causes stiffness – and, therefore, added pain – but also interferes with sleep. TV provokes numerous emotional responses in rapid succession. It quickens the heart rate and releases chemicals (such as adrenaline) for no useful purpose. When these chemicals are produced naturally, we deal with the situation and blood flow is returned to normal. However, when chemicals are induced second-hand, by watching TV, they remain in the bloodstream. This causes tension to linger and, ultimately, gives rise to more pain.

Keeping warm

As we well know, cold has an adverse effect in fibromyalgia. Sitting in a draught can cause our muscles to stiffen and our pain levels to rise and standing at a bus stop in a bitterly cold wind can provoke a severe flare-up. Although we don't always do what is best for us, we soon learn to avoid such situations. When we take steps to keep warm at all times, wrapping up when we go outside and ensuring we stay warm, too, indoors, muscle flexibility is encouraged.

Direct application of heat usually releases muscle tension. It increases blood flow through the tissues, encouraging oxygenation and removing toxins. Direct heat can come in the form of warm showers or baths, infra-red heating lamps, microwavable wheat bags, electric under- and over-blankets, hot water bottles, electric heating pads and muscle-warming massage cream.

The use of cold

Trigger points or other painful areas are often more responsive to the application of cold than they are to heat. Placed directly over a painful area, an ice-pack, for example, can moderate the transmission of pain messages to the CNS. (The ice-pack, bag of frozen peas or refrigerator-cooled wheat bag should never be placed directly on the skin but wrapped in a tea towel.) A routine of ten minutes on, then ten minutes off is recommended.

Relaxing the muscles

When we are anxious or in pain, we subconsciously tighten our muscles, which causes more pain. It is important, therefore, that people with fibromyalgia learn to recognize increasing tenseness and make efforts to check involuntary tightening.

The technique of tightening and then relaxing different muscle groups is not recommended in fibromyalgia. The mere act of tightening can give rise to pain that is not easy to shift.

Action for flare-ups

Flare-ups of pain are an ever present risk in fibromyalgia. They can be caused by:

- the physical stress of repetitive work;
- emotional stress and/or insomnia;
- a fall or bump;
- cold and/or damp weather conditions;
- hormonal changes brought about by the menstrual cycle.

When a person makes no attempt to manage the pain of a flare-up, his or her condition may rapidly deteriorate. This can create feelings of anger and despair which, in turn, increases pain. Unless the following factors are carefully observed, the situation can become very difficult.

Self-help plan for flare-ups

1 Recognize when your pain levels are rising. Take action before it gets worse. This may include immediate rest, application of heat or cold, painkilling/muscle-relaxing medication, massage, myofascial (trigger-point) release therapy, aromatherapy treatment, relaxation and meditation exercises, use of a TENS machine or whatever works best for you.

2 Be positive! A positive frame of mind speeds recovery. Tell yourself, 'I'll get through this just as I have before', 'I am more aware of how to help myself this time', 'I'll make efforts to distract myself', 'I won't let myself get depressed. I know that does more harm than good.'

3 Explore the possible reasons for the increase in pain. Ask yourself, 'Did I overexert myself?', 'Did I forget to pace myself?', 'Should I have driven the car when I was already feeling fragile?', 'Did I sit in one position for too long?', 'Was I leaning forward too much?'

4 Decide how you can reduce the risk of future flare-ups. Do this by asking for help when you need it, being clearer about what you can and can't do and aligning your expectations of yourself and others with what is practicable. All of these are helpful emotionally as well as physically.

5 Review the effectiveness of your current flare-up strategy. Is your present medication adequate in a crisis? Can you do anything further to help you stay positive? Is it time to visit your doctor again? Could you try a new type of complementary therapy?

Other points to review

- *Sleep and rest* Because of the link between fibromyalgia and sleep, do try and get more sleep, by means of either an earlier bedtime or a lie-in. If like many people with fibromyalgia you have difficulty sleeping, you may find that more time relaxing, especially in the afternoon, may help. It may seem counter-intuitive, but wearing yourself out with exercise doesn't always make for sound, restful sleep. For a stressed, sensitized system, it may be more helpful to spend time after lunch listening to music, meditating (see page 159), having a hot bath or just resting. Go lightly on the exercise – maybe try a modified version of your usual routine, without abandoning it altogether.

- *Medication* If you are experiencing a lot of flare-ups, talk to your doctor about your current level and type of medication.
- *Diet* Review your diet, particularly your intake of sugar, white unrefined flour and processed foods and ready-meals. A cleansing day of fresh fruit and vegetables, with some light protein such as lentils, may help.
- *Water intake* Ensure you are drinking enough water, preferably eight glasses a day, either plain or by means of juices, herbal teas, ice lollies, and so on.
- *Stress* Avoid upset and confrontation as much as possible. Learn to say no. Let family, friends and work colleagues get on without you for a day or so – you can make it up to them when you feel stronger.

Stress management

Stress arises not only as a result of what happens to us, but also from our reactions to these things. Negative attitudes can actually cause people to see catastrophe in what to others would be normal, everyday events. When a situation is interpreted as a crisis, adrenaline is released into the bloodstream and the body automatically puts itself 'on alert'. Breathing becomes shallow and fast, the heart rate quickens, blood pressure rises and the muscles tense, allowing the individual to deal with an emergency more effectively. These responses can be destructive, however, when they occur frequently.

Delay your reaction

Because living with a chronic pain condition naturally creates stress in daily life, people with fibromyalgia experience higher levels of stress than do people without it. However, curbing your responses to certain occurrences can greatly reduce stress build-up and the incidence of flare-ups. As a troublesome event unfolds, try not to react instantly. By postponing your response, you allow yourself time to evaluate the situation, to see it as it really is. Now select a response that doesn't create more stress.

Self-talk

The way we speak to ourselves has great bearing on our stress levels. When we analyse our thoughts, we are often surprised at their negativity, but they must be examined before we can begin to change their destructive pattern. When the TV breaks down, for example, your initial thoughts may be, 'It's so unfair! I was really looking forward to watching that film!', 'This is all I need! I can't afford a new TV!', 'Even if it can be repaired, it will probably cost a small fortune!', 'What am I supposed to do with my time – sit twiddling my thumbs?' – stress-provoking thoughts by any standard!

By being aware that negative thoughts create stress, you can train yourself into more positive self-talk. Using the same example, you may, instead, think, 'I'll ring around for quotes in the morning. Maybe it won't cost much to repair', 'It was on its last legs anyway. I'll take the opportunity to buy a more up-to-date TV', 'I could buy a new TV on a 0 per cent hire-purchase deal', 'I could buy a reconditioned TV if I can't afford a new one', 'I could rent one and not have to worry about repair costs', 'I wonder if my friend down the road is watching that film?' or 'In the meantime, this is my chance to read that book, finish my tapestry, phone Aunt Betty ...'

The following examples of stress-relieving self-talk can be applied to many potentially stressful situations.

> 'I'll break this problem into separate sections. They'll be easier to handle.'
> 'I'll take things one step at a time.'
> 'Is this really worth getting upset and angry over?'
> 'I've coped before, so I'll cope again.'
> 'I can always ask for help if I need it.'
> 'It could have been much worse.'
> 'This is hardly a matter of life or death!'
> 'There's nothing I can do about this situation, so I'll have to accept it.'

Life stress evaluation

If you take time to evaluate all the relationships and activities in your everyday life, you are likely to find that some prompt more stress than benefit. Fibromyalgia demands that you protect your body and nourish your mind. 'Involvements' that have ceased to do this are probably harmful.

In reviewing your relationships and activities, however, remember that personal interactions and energy-related performances will always produce a certain amount of stress. It is when the stress outweighs the positive gains that you need to consider limiting or ceasing your involvement in them.

Address your stress

1 *List aspects of looking after the home that cause stress.* Taking each problem in turn, can you make things easier for yourself? For example, you could try asking for help, share the housework, accept that you will have an untidier house in future.
2 *List the stressful aspects of your job.* How can you make these things less stressful? For example, you could inform your boss and co-workers of your limitations, not place yourself under pressure, reduce your hours, find less taxing employment.
3 *List personal relationships that are particularly stressful.* Taking each in turn, how exactly can you improve the situation? For example, could you express your needs and feelings more clearly, lower your expectations of the person(s) in question, limit your interactions with such people?
4 *List the organizations, societies or groups that create more stress than benefit.* Remember that partaking in group activities can be diverting, uplifting and give you a real sense of purpose. Try to be honest about whether the stress really does outweigh the gains. If there is truly a problem, how exactly can you improve the situation? Perhaps you could inform the person in charge that you need to limit your duties, take on a different, perhaps more rewarding, role, take a break from your involvement for a period, end your association with the organization.

Chronic stress

Chronic stress is the state of being constantly 'on alert'. The physiological changes associated with this state – a fast heart rate, shallow breathing and muscle tension – persist over a long period, making relaxation difficult. Chronic stress can lead to nerviness, hypertension, irritability and depression.

The condition commonly arises when any of the following needs fail to be met on a long-term basis.

- *The need to be understood*
Although this subject has been discussed earlier in this chapter, I will reiterate that people with fibromyalgia long to talk truthfully about how they feel and be taken at their word. Being misunderstood can induce frustration, irritability and despondency. Feelings of helplessness (you cannot change other people's minds) and isolation (you learn not to expect to be understood) may arise too, causing you to shut others out. However, it is not easy for others to accept and understand, particularly when your illness affects their needs. Sharing your feelings without blaming anyone is the most important step towards being understood.

- *The need to be loved*
Feeling unloveable is doubtless the greatest threat to the emotional well-being of people with fibromyalgia. You may tell yourself you have more to worry about than your appearance, yet feel concern that your partner now finds you unattractive and so will ultimately end the relationship, and this may make you subconsciously withdraw your affections. You may wonder how anyone *could* love you the way you are looking, for you may have developed 'pain lines' around your eyes and mouth, you may have dark shadows beneath your eyes and, due to inactivity, you may have put on weight. You may even have become miserable, irrational and antagonistic. Moreover, you doubt anyone could really love someone with chronic pain, who would severely limit life.

  Before you can be loved by others, you need to love yourself. You need to see yourself as a worthwhile person with qualities that you, as well as others, can respect. Don't let apathy rule. Start the way you mean to go on by doing the following:
  - make a list of your ten best attributes;
  - do one nice thing (however small) for another person each day, and don't forget to congratulate yourself for doing it;
  - make the most of your appearance, within your physical and financial scope;
  - regularly treat yourself to something uplifting – an aromatherapy or reflexology massage, for example;
  - try to frequently indulge in something that stimulates your mind as well as creating a sense of fulfilment.

- *The need to love*
  Fibromyalgia can cause introversion. It can cause you to wholly
  focus on your symptoms, ultimately withdrawing from those
  around you. However, loving others and actively attempting
  to cheer them can have a positive impact on your own life. For
  example, encouraging your partner to smile can lift your own
  mood, phoning a friend with relationship problems can make
  you feel useful and having a nice chat with a lonely neighbour
  can hearten you both.

  Where pleasing others is concerned, a careful balance must be
  sought, however. People with fibromyalgia are often inclined to
  put others first. Saying 'yes' to a request to collect young Lizzie
  from school because her mum is doing some decorating can, if
  you are having a bad day yourself, be counter-productive. As well
  as being angry with yourself for overdoing it, you may also feel
  used. Lizzie's mum is more able than you. She could have picked
  the child up herself.

  In giving to others, you must be careful not to exceed your
  limitations. You can make someone smile with a few carefully
  chosen words and a bit of honest flattery will make you feel
  just as good as the recipient. Instead of being defensive around
  others, try to understand their needs. They will likely be pleased
  and uplifted by the effort you have made and, hopefully, will
  want to respond in kind. You have to give before you can hope
  to receive.

- *The need to achieve*
  Although the subject of 'achievement' has been discussed earlier
  in this chapter, I will just add here that, in general, we are happy
  when we are producing something, when we feel we are of value.
  To be unproductive creates boredom and restlessness and giving
  up fulfilling activities breeds doubts about ever again experiencing feelings of achievement. However, those feelings really
  can be regained when, in accepting our limits, we carefully pace
  activities previously enjoyed or, alternatively, take up rewarding
  substitute activities.

- *The need to be supported*
  As personal 'support' was covered earlier in this chapter, I just
  want to say here that people with fibromyalgia need the emotional and physical backing of others. Asking for help can feel

humiliating, especially when we are used to priding ourselves on our capabilities. When we refuse to request assistance, however, we can get upset about others failing to second-guess our needs and we fret about the effects of doing too much ourselves. In order to avoid these negative emotions, do ask and try not to make the mistake of being unappreciative when others lend a hand. Accept help with good grace and your stress levels will automatically drop.

- *The need to be yourself*
  The roles many of us play out, perhaps unawares, often, as we saw earlier, have their origins in early childhood. If, for example, the parents of young Carl were scathing of incompetence when he was growing up, he may prize competence himself into adulthood, going so far as to hide instances when he is less than perfect. Only when he moves in with a partner who is far from perfect, a partner who is maybe even intimidated by Carl's apparent 'perfection', will he begin to see that it is all right to be flawed.

  There may be several ways in which you hide your real self. You may, for example, have been out with a person who lived and breathed football. You liked him a lot so you read the sports pages and feigned interest. However, realistically, going through life pretending to be interested in something you don't actually care a lot about causes untold stress. It is far better to be yourself for, apart from minimizing stress, you also know that the people important to you like you for who you really are.

- *The need to feel well*
  Constantly feeling unwell is perhaps the most forbidding aspect of fibromyalgia. However, we can, as we find our feet, take steps to lessen the awareness of illness, as well as the severity of the condition itself. For instance, we can eat healthily, take regular (careful) exercise, avoid the foods and other substances to which we know we are sensitive, forge satisfactory relationships with our doctors, families and friends, learn the art of positive thinking and try different complementary therapies. Whether or not the benefits are only temporary, the feeling that we are actively helping ourselves creates a sense of achievement. In addition, activities that challenge the mind can help reduce feelings of uselessness and are fundamental to building self-esteem. They also lower stress levels.

When essential needs are not met

For people with fibromyalgia, meeting these seven essential needs is far from easy. People with the condition may be neither understood, nor supported, so they feel unloveable, fear they have little to offer others, feel devalued and that their achievements are limited and rarely feel well. Against such odds, the road ahead is undeniably bumpy. However, knowing your emotional needs – and endeavouring to meet them – will undoubtedly have a positive effect on your pain and stress levels.

Relaxation techniques

Fibromyalgia is a condition for which medical science can, at present, do very little. Although experts by no means advocate that we should 'grin and bear' the pain, it is advisable that fibromyalgia-related medication be used as sparingly as possible, given individual circumstances. People with fibromyalgia achieve most success by means of self-help, many forms of which have been outlined earlier. However, the purest forms of self-help are deep breathing, relaxation and meditation – all natural therapies you can do yourself.

Deep breathing

In normal breathing, we take oxygen from the atmosphere down into our lungs. The diaphragm contracts – and air is pulled into the chest cavity. When we breathe out, we expel carbon dioxide and other waste gases back into the atmosphere. However, when we are stressed or upset, or just from habit, we tend to use the rib muscles to expand the chest, breathing more quickly, sucking in air and breathing it out shallowly. This is good in a crisis as it allows us to obtain the optimum amount of oxygen in the shortest possible time, providing our bodies with the extra power needed to handle the emergency.

Some people do tend to get stuck in shallow, chest-breathing mode. In the long term, shallow breathing is not only detrimental to our physical and emotional health, it can also lead to hyperventilation, panic attacks, chest pains, dizziness and gastrointestinal problems.

To test your breathing, ask yourself the following questions.

- How fast are you breathing as you read this?
- Are you pausing between breaths?
- Are you breathing with your chest or with your diaphragm?

A deep breathing exercise

The following deep breathing exercise should, ideally, be performed daily.

1 Make yourself comfortable, lying down in a warm room where you know you will be undisturbed for at least half an hour.
2 Close your eyes and try to relax.
3 Gradually slow down your breathing, inhaling and exhaling as evenly as possible.
4 Place one hand on your chest and the other on your abdomen, just below your ribcage.
5 As you inhale steadily and slowly through your nose, allow your abdomen to swell upwards – your chest should barely move.
6 As you exhale steadily and slowly through your mouth, let your abdomen flatten – empty your lungs completely.

Give yourself a few minutes to get into a smooth, easy rhythm. As worries and distractions arise, don't hang on to them – wait calmly for them to float out of your mind, then focus once more on your breathing.

When you feel ready to end the exercise, open your eyes. Allow yourself time to become alert before rolling over on to one side and getting up. With practice, you will start to breathe with your diaphragm quite naturally all the time and in times of stress, you should be able to correct your breathing without too much effort.

Deep relaxation

Relaxation is one of the forgotten skills in today's hectic world. We already know that stress – which can give rise to muscle tension, insomnia, hypertension and depression – is perhaps the greatest enemy of a person with fibromyalgia. It is advisable, therefore, to learn at least one relaxation technique. The following exercise is perhaps the easiest.

A deep relaxation exercise

1 Make yourself comfortable in a place where you will not be disturbed – listening to restful music may help you relax.

2 Begin to slow down your breathing, inhaling steadily and slowly through your nose for a count of two, ensuring that the abdomen pushes outwards as you breathe in (as explained in the deep breathing exercise above).

3 Now exhale slowly and steadily through your mouth for a count of four, five or six.

4 After a couple of minutes, concentrate on each part of the body in turn, starting with your right arm. Consciously relax each set of muscles, allowing the tension to flow right out. Let your arm feel heavier and heavier as every last remnant of tension seeps away. Follow this procedure with the muscles of your left arm, then the muscles of your face, neck, stomach, hips and, finally, your legs and feet.

Visualization

When you have reached step 4 of the deep relaxation exercise above, visualization can be introduced. As you continue to breathe slowly and evenly, imagine yourself surrounded, perhaps, by lush, peaceful countryside, beside a gently trickling stream or maybe on a deserted tropical beach, beneath swaying palm fronds, listening to the sounds of the ocean, thousands of miles from your worries and cares. Let the warm sun, the gentle breeze, the peacefulness of it all wash over you.

The tranquillity you feel at this stage can be enhanced by frequently repeating the exercise – once or twice a day is best. With time, you should be able to switch into a calm state of mind whenever you feel stressed. I will reiterate that relaxed muscles use far less energy than tense ones and that improved breathing leads to better circulation and oxygenation – which, in turn, helps the muscles and connective tissues. A relaxed mind can also greatly aid concentration and short-term memory. It can help eliminate 'brain fog', too. All positive benefits, I'm sure you'll agree!

Meditation

Arguably the oldest natural therapy, meditation is the simplest and most effective form of self-help. Ideally, you should initially be taught the technique by a teacher but, as meditation is essentially performed alone, it can be learned alone with equal success.

The unusual thing about meditation is that it involves 'letting go', allowing the mind to roam freely. However, as most of us are used to striving to control our thoughts, letting go is not so easy as it sounds.

It may help to know that people who regularly meditate say they have more energy, require less sleep, are less anxious and feel far 'more alive' than before they did so. Studies have shown that, during meditation, the heartbeat slows, blood pressure lowers and circulation improves, making the hands and feet feel much warmer.

Meditation may, to some people, sound a bit off-beat, something hippies do, but isn't it worth a try – especially when you can do it for free? Kick off those shoes and make yourself comfortable, somewhere you can be undisturbed for a while. Now follow these simple instructions.

First steps in meditation

1 Close your eyes, relax and practise the deep breathing exercise described above.
2 Concentrate on your breathing. Try to free your mind of conscious control. Letting it roam unchecked, try to allow the deeper, more serene part of you to take over.
3 If you wish to go further into meditation, concentrate now on mentally repeating a 'mantra', which is a certain word or phrase. It should be something positive such as 'relax', 'I feel calm', 'I am feeling much better' or 'I am special', whatever works best for you.
4 When you are ready to finish, open your eyes and allow yourself time to adjust to the outside world before getting to your feet.

The aim of mentally or actually repeating a mantra out loud is to plant the positive thought into your subconscious mind. It is a form of self-hypnosis and only you control the messages placed there.

Useful addresses

General

FibroAction
Tel.: 0844 443 5422
Website: www.fibroaction.org

This charitable organization provides information about fibromyalgia, and has a good social media team to help and support people, mainly online.

The Fibromyalgia Association UK
Studio 3007, Mile End Mill
12 Seedhill Road
Paisley PA1 1JS
Tel.: 0844 826 9022 (general enquiries, not for support)
Helpline: 0844 887 2444 (10 a.m. to 4 p.m., Monday to Friday)
Website: www.fmauk.org

A registered charity administered by volunteers and established to provide information and support to those with the condition and their families. In addition the Association provides medical information for professionals, a patient-information pack and a magazine, *Fibromyalgia Focus*. The website contains a community forum.

Fibromyalgia Support Northern Ireland
PO Box 293
Bangor BT20 9AQ
Tel.: 028 9127 1525
Helpline: 0844 826 9024 (10.30 a.m. to 4 p.m., Monday to Friday)
Text: 08448 269024 (for urgent enquiries when out and about: no abbreviations please)
Website: www.fmsni.org.uk

This organization is dedicated to raising fibromyalgia awareness and supporting people with fibromyalgia. Drop-in services are available in Belfast and Coleraine.

National Fibromyalgia Association
1000 Bristol Street, North Suite 17–247,
Newport Beach
CA 92660
USA
Website: www.fmaware.org

The members-only website provides an online store and chatroom and gives information on support groups and FM community events from Canada to California. The monthly *Fibromyalgia AWARE* magazine (at present *The New! Fibromyalgia AWARE Magazine*) may be received online or in a printed version by subscription.

UK Fibromyalgia
7 Ashbourne Road
Bournemouth BH5 2JS
Tel. and Fax: 01202 259155
Website: www.ukfibromyalgia.com

For fibromyalgia information and advice, experts' comments and more. Providers of the monthly *Fibromyalgia* magazine.

Legal

Andrew Isaacs Solicitors Ltd
Richmond House
White Rose Way
Doncaster
South Yorkshire DN4 5JH
Tel.: 01302 349480
Website: www.andrewisaacs.co.uk

For information and advice regarding possible litigation claims.

Brian Barr Solicitors
Grosvenor House
Off Agecroft Road
Manchester M27 8UW
Tel.: 0161 737 9248
Fax: 0161 637 4946
Website: www.brianbarr.co.uk

Mr Barr is familiar with fibromyalgia and has represented those with the condition in making successful claims.

Seasonal affective disorder (SAD)

Outside In (Cambridge) Ltd
Unit 31, Dry Drayton Estate
Scotland Road
Cambridge CB3 8AT
Tel.: 01954 211955/0845 658 9292
Website: www.outsidein.co.uk

Suppliers of a variety of light-therapy products.

SAD-Shop
16 Stanley Street
Southport PR9 0BY
Tel.: 01704 500505 (advice hotline)
Website: www.sad-lighthire.co.uk

Lightboxes used to treat SAD can be hired or bought from this company.

Seasonal Affective Disorder Association (SADA)
PO Box 332
Wallingford
Oxon OX10 1EP
Website: www.sada.org.uk

A voluntary organization and registered charity which informs the public and health professions about seasonal affective disorder and supports and advises those with the condition.

Other organizations

Arthritis Care
Floor 4, Linen Court
10 East Road
London N1 6AD
Tel.: 020 7380 6500
Helpline: 0808 800 4050 (free, 10 a.m. to 4 p.m., Monday to Friday)
Website: www.arthritiscare.org.uk

The website provides details of other regional and national offices in the UK.

Arthritis Research UK
Copeman House
St Mary's Court
St Mary's Gate
Chesterfield S41 7TD
Tel.: 0300 790 0400
Website: www.arthritisresearchuk.org

Association of Reflexologists
5 Fore Street
Taunton
Somerset TA1 1HX
Tel.: 01823 351010
Website: www.aor.org.uk

Backcare
The Old Office Block
16 Elmtree Road
Teddington
Middlesex TW11 8ST
Tel.: 020 8977 5474
Helpline: 0845 130 2704
Website: www.backcare.org.uk

The Bowen Association
PO Box 210
Boston PE21 1DD
Tel.: 01205 319100
Email: office@bowen-technique.co.uk

British Acupuncture Council
63 Jeddo Road
London W12 9HQ
Tel.: 020 8735 0400 (9.30 a.m. to 5.30 p.m., Monday to Friday)
Website: www.acupuncture.org.uk

British Chiropractic Association
59 Castle Street
Reading
Berkshire RG1 7SN
Tel.: 0118 950 5950 (9 a.m. to 5 p.m., Monday to Friday)
Website: www.chiropractic-uk.co.uk

British Homeopathic Association
Hahnemann House
29 Park Street West
Luton LU1 3BE
Tel.: 01582 408675
Website: www.britishhomeopathic.org

Carers UK
20 Great Dover Street
London SE1 4LX
Tel.: 020 7378 4999
Helpline: 0808 808 7777 (10 a.m. to 4 p.m., Monday to Friday)
Website: www.carersuk.org

Carers UK is the voice of carers. The association gives support to those who provide unpaid care by looking after an ill, frail or disabled family member, friend or partner.

Further reading

Dr Megan Arroll, *Chronic Fatigue Syndrome: What You Need to Know About CFS/ME*, Sheldon Press, London, 2014

Stacie L. Bigelow, *Fibromyalgia: Simple Relief Through Movement*, John Wiley & Sons, London, 2000

Christine Craggs-Hinton, *Fibromyalgia: Your Treatment Guide*, Overcoming Common Problems, Sheldon Press, London, 2013

Christine Craggs-Hinton, *The Fibromyalgia Healing Diet*, Overcoming Common Problems, third edition, Sheldon Press, London, 2014

Christine Craggs-Hinton, *How to Beat Pain: Pain Relief Techniques That Work*, Overcoming Common Problems, Sheldon Press, London, 2005

Claudia Craig Marek, *The First Year: Fibromyalgia – A Patient-expert Guide for the Newly Diagnosed*, Robinson Publishing, London, 2004

Patricia Davis, *Aromatherapy: An A–Z: The Most Comprehensive Guide to Aromatherapy Ever*, Vermilion, London, 2005

Dr Kristina Downing-Orr, *Beating Chronic Fatigue: Your Step-by-step Guide to Complete Recovery*, Piatkus, London, 2013

Joe Fitzgibbon, *Feeling Tired All the Time*, Gill and Macmillan, London, 2001

Wendy Green, *50 Things You Can Do to Manage Fibromyalgia*, Summersdale Publishing, Chichester, 2012

Professor John Hunter, *Irritable Bowel Solutions: The Essential Guide to IBS, its Causes and Treatments*, Vermilion, London, 2007

Harris H. McIlwain and Debra Fulghum Bruce, *The Fibromyalgia Handbook: A 7-Step Program to Halt and Even Reverse Fibromyalgia*, Saint Martin's Press Inc., London, 2003

Neville Shone, *Coping Successfully with Pain*, Overcoming Common Problems, Sheldon Press, London, 2002

Shelly Ann Smith, *The Fibromyalgia Cookbook: More Than 120 Easy and Delicious Recipes*, Cumberland House Publishing, Nashville, TN, 2002

Roland Staud MD and Christine Adamec, *Fibromyalgia for Dummies*, John Wiley & Sons, London, 2007

Erica Verrillo, *Chronic Fatigue Syndrome: A Treatment Guide*, second edition (Kindle), 2012

Index

activities and lifestyle, adjusting
   60–9, 132–4; driving 67–8; lifting
   and carrying 64–7; reaching up 64;
   rising from a chair 68; shopping
   134; typing 62–3; washing-up 64
acupressure 89
acupuncture 5, 25, 88, 89–90, 105
allergies 2, 14, 15, 25–6, 51
anti-convulsants 37
antidepressants 13, 16, 29, 36, 57,
   69, 100
anxiety 12, 14, 15, 18, 20–1, 37, 54,
   56, 57, 91, 100
aromatherapy 88, 90, 105
arthritis 5, 12, 35, 53, 142

Bach flower remedies 93–4
bioelectromagnetics 95–6
Bowen technique 96

caffeine 20, 21, 30, 44, 49, 57
candida albicans 22, 45–6
carers 112
central nervous system (CNS) 7, 8, 9,
   10, 11, 142, 145, 148
central sensitization 7–9
cervical stenosis 8
chemical sensitivity 25–6
chiropractic 97–8
coenzyme Q10 52–3
cognitive behavioural therapy 14
cognitive dysfunction ('foggy brain')
   2, 15, 27–8
cold, use of 27, 148
complementary therapies 88–109
cooling-down exercises *see under*
   exercises
crisis medication 144–5

depression 2, 12, 15, 16, 19–20, 56,
   100
diagnosis 13
diet ch. 4; recommendations 43–4
digestive system ch. 4
distraction 143–4

dorsal horn 8
driving *see under* activities and
   lifestyle, adjusting
dry eyes and mouth (sicca syndrome)
   15, 29

endocrine system (hormones) 6, 42,
   100
endorphins 81, 109, 132, 143, 145
environmental toxins 6
epidural anaesthetics 38
exercise 69–71; *see also* ch. 5
exercises ch. 5; aerobic 81–2; aqua-
   aerobics 83–4; cooling-down 84–6;
   cycling 84; mobility 73–4; stepping
   83; strengthening 77–81; stretching
   59, 71, 75–7; trampoline 83;
   treadmill 68; walking 82; warm-up
   47, 58–61, 72

fatigue 2, 6, 15, 16–18
fear 112–13
fine nerve abnormalities *see* nerve
   abnormalities
food elimination programme 48–51

ginkgo biloba 99–100
guaifenesin 39–41
guilt 110, 112, 117
Gulf War syndrome 26
gut microflora 22, 45–6; permeability
   47–8

headaches 24–5, 46, 100
herbal remedies 98–101
homeopathy 101–2
hormonal imbalances 6
hydrotherapy 102
hypnotherapy 103–4
hypoglycaemia 17, 43, 48

immune system 6, 23, 26, 42, 45–7,
   53, 92
irrational feelings 119–22
irritable bladder 28

irritable bowel syndrome (IBS) 21–4

jaw pain *see* temperomandibular joint (TMJ) dysfunction

lifting and carrying *see under* activities and lifestyle, adjusting
light therapy 17
lignocaine infusions 39
lying down for long periods 67

massage 104–5
medication ch. 3
meditation 159
microcurrent stimulation 97
microtraumas (muscle tears) 3, 27, 70, 72
migraines 25, 46, 100
mood swings 14, 17
morning stiffness 28, 108
MRI (Magnetic Resonance Imaging) scans 8
muscle: relaxants 37, 144; spasms 15, 27, 34, 35, 36, 37; tension 4
music therapy 108–9
myalgic encephalomyelitis (ME) 17
myofascial pain syndrome (MPS) 3, 5

narcotic analgesia 34–5
neck injury/trauma 7, 8; *see also* whiplash injury
negative thinking 118–22
nerve abnormalities 2, 6, 7, 9, 11–12, 30
neurotransmitters 143
nocturnal myoclonus 29–30
non-steroidal anti-inflammatory drugs (NSAIDs) 35
numbness and tingling (paresthesia) 30

osteoporosis 2, 31–2, 82

pain: circuitry 10; filtering mechanisms 8; management ch. 7; messages 9, 10, 11, 148; origins of 3–4; process 10, 11; widespread 2–3
painkillers 13, 24, 33–6; natural 81, 143
panic attacks 21

paroxetine 16
peripheral neuropathy *see* nerve abnormalities
pet therapy 109
post-traumatic malfunction 8
posture 4, ch. 5
Prozac 16, 100

reflexology 106
rehabilitation programmes 12
relaxation ch. 7
restless leg syndrome 29

St John's wort 100
seasonal affective disorder (SAD) 16–17
selective serotonin re-uptake inhibitors (SSRIs) 16
serotonin 6, 9, 16, 17, 52, 56, 100
sertraline 16
skin problems 13, 30
sleep 6, 11, 15, 18–19, 145–8
small fibre peripheral neuropathy (SFPN) 11
spinal abnormalities 8–9
stress management 3, 4, 5, 7, 21, 24, 25, 30, 44, ch. 7
substance P 9
supplements *see* vitamins and minerals

temperomandibular joint (TMJ) dysfunction/jaw pain 27
tender points 4, 13, 107
Transcutaneous Electrical Nerve Stimulation (TENS) machines 145
trigger points 3, 4–5, 27, 148, 149; injections 38

ultrasound 97

visualization 158
vitamin D 53–4
vitamins and minerals 32, 49, 51–6
vulnerability, feelings of 111

whiplash injury 7, 8, 69

yeast: allergy 47; toxins 46–7
yoga 106–8